Teach Kind, Clear Yoga

A GUIDE FOR PRACTITIONERS AND TEACHERS

Kathryn Anne Flynn

The information provided in this book is designed to provide helpful informa-tion on the subjects within and is not in any manner a substitute for medical advice. For diagnosis or treatment of any health or medical issue, consult your own healthcare provider.

The author assumes no responsibility or liability for any injuries or negative consequences that arise from following the information in this book. Always consult with a healthcare provider before embarking on a yoga practice or any other exercise program.

Reference is provided for informational purposes only and does not consti-tute an endorsement of any websites or other sources. Readers should be aware that any websites referred to in this book may change.

ISBN 978-1-7774031-0-2 (Paperback edition)
ISBN 978-1-7774031-1-9 (ePub edition)

Editor: Lesley-Anne Longo
Cover and book design: Nicole Madison
Pose photos: Fitch Jean
Headshot photo: Rémi Thériault

To Bernice, and to the memories of Margaret and Harvey.
You taught me how to love well.

Contents

Foreword

WHEN I TOOK MY very first yoga teacher training in 2003, there were lots of yoga books. Still, not many yoga books that explained teaching methodology to support new teachers. Given how many people sign up for yoga teacher training (perhaps you might be one of them?), an obvious need arose in the yoga community.

Each yoga teacher training program is unique and has specific focuses based on its facilitators' understanding and abilities – never mind the lineage or style of yoga they emphasize. Most YTT (yoga teacher training) programs provide a manual to their students for reference. Few of these manuals are meant or available for reading outside of the program. Given that a foundational YTT is typically about 200 hours in length (which is not a very long time) and that all humans have blind spots, it is fair to put on the table that any given program likely has a blind spot or two of its own. Please do not mistake my comment as being derogatory towards yoga teacher training programs – I run two YTTs myself – it is more an acknowledgement of the reality of the context in which YTTs occur. We are all doing our best, with what we know, and the time we have.

As I write this foreword in the year 2020, many books exist on yoga, which makes good sense given how vast a science and technology yoga is and its great interest. This book, Teach Kind, Clear Yoga, is a welcome addition to the newly growing section of books on approaches to yoga teaching methodology. Yes, there is information on technique. However, Kathryn takes time to explain and articulate the importance of creating yoga environments that honor a wide variety of practitioners' abilities and capacities, all while highlighting the importance of considering what we are doing as teachers and why.

This thoughtfully written book offers information and practical advice. It also provides important contemplations and exercises to support your growth and development as a yoga and yoga teacher *asana*. This book also gives lovely tangible ways to actually bring kindness, a form of *ahimsa*, into your classes. Then it isn't just something you talk about, but rather something you practice with your students and invite them to practice through their yoga experiences. I am reminded of Brené Brown in her book Dare to Lead - *"Clear is kind, unclear is unkind"*. Being able to approach teaching this way is much needed.

Knowing Kathryn, I can also appreciate that her fabulous sense of humor and personality are part of the package. This makes the read enjoyable, and I spent a lot of time smiling as I read, as I am sure you will as well.

So whether you are considering taking a yoga teacher training, or have already taken one, this book is filled with information and ideas that will support you to teach to a wide variety of students, to create communal environments in your classes, and to take a practical approach to how you deliver classes. If you're holding this book in your hands, you have taken a wise step in a fruitful direction. Congratulations, and let the learning begin!

with peace & love,
Mona L. Warner
November 2020

Introduction

DO YOU REMEMBER WHY you started practicing yoga? Was it to ease your lower back pain? Reduce stress? Or did you just need something to do on Wednesday evenings and a reason to wear stretchy clothes?

Yoga practice typically begins with immediate needs in the hope of relief. Many people start yoga to manage their stress levels or reduce physical pain, but find their yoga practice evolves into profound psychological calm and broadening feelings of goodwill. Yoga can be a practice of spiritual and ethical inquiry, and our openness to these limbs of yoga can be surprising when remembering our initial goals.

I started practicing yoga because I suffered a terrible knee injury at 21 as a result of poor running form and ignoring my body's warning signs that something was wrong, like painful shin splints. I felt like I needed to run to lose weight, be slim, and obtain happiness, so I endured the pain until it literally knocked me off my feet. I could barely climb the stairs and, most tragically, had to wear "practical shoes" (i.e., old lady shoes) to my university graduation.

My mother, who had been teaching yoga for a few years at this point, encouraged me to attend yoga classes. I resisted until she said the magic words: "Would you take some private classes if I *paid for them*?" I started my one-on-one classes that week, in a tiny local studio with a woman who seemed to know everything about how to use a tennis ball to relieve hip tension, plus the secrets of the universe, too. I was awed, and I was hooked.

Practicing yoga got me out of pain and back into movement; it also became a tool for managing harmful mental states like the one that had me running myself into injury.

This tiny summary of the beginning of my yoga journey in no way captures the enormity of what yoga has done for me. Sometimes it's hard not to sound a little cheesy talking about our relationship with yoga, because of the depth of personal meaning it carries.

When yoga practitioners feel their lives are positively transformed by practices that are largely accessible, or they want to evolve their relationship with yoga, they may choose to take yoga teacher training.

Yoga's popularity has changed the yoga classroom at all levels. A 2013 study estimated that 250 million people are actively practicing[1] around the world, drawing people of all ethnicities, body types, ages, and accessibility levels. The yoga classroom is becoming more diverse, a process generated by its increasing popularity and efforts from some individuals seeking to improve accessibility.

This book is for yoga teachers who teach the "general population," loosely defined as folks who are practicing yoga for general wellness. They likely have little or no attachment to some of yoga's athletic postural accomplishments, like Headstand (*Sirsasana)* and Wheel pose (*Chakrasana)*, but would like to be in less physical and/or emotional/mental pain. They can get down onto the ground to be on a yoga mat and get back up to get into standing postures, but rapidly changing between standing postures and other postures may pose a challenge.

Excellent physical fitness is not a prerequisite for a yoga class when you design yoga sequences for the general population. For example, when planning our classes, we should keep in mind that 25% of Canadians between the ages of 50–64 have high blood pressure.[2] We might remember that 63.1% of Canadians have a body weight classified as a health risk (i.e., overweight or obese).[3] We could consider that people internalize the pressure to be in better physical shape, even as their workplaces, life demands, and healthcare systems are unsupportive of preventive health measures.

So instead of making our classes about fitness experiences alone, we endeavor to offer experiences of accessible movement, a break from our hyperconnected world, and a space for compassionate self-inquiry.

The average folks who make up the new yoga student body are becoming our yoga teachers. Foundational yoga teacher training programs are flourishing, and have become essential yoga education. Even in my time as a yoga teacher trainer, the students in the program are increasingly "typical" folks—not "typical yoga folks." I've had teacher trainees of all ages—one as young as 19, to one "chronologically experienced" trainee of 75 years of age. At every information session I have offered for a foundational yoga program, it's inevitable that someone worriedly asks about the importance of advanced yoga postures as a prerequisite to entry. Each time, I reassure the trainee that practicing or teaching headstands is not a prerequisite for yoga teacher training, or for a healthy, happy life.

The average yoga teacher is not what the media portrays. Popular impressions of yoga teachers are consistently white, young women with circus-performer levels of flexibility and an abundance of time for self-care. When I think of the average yoga teacher these days, I think of "Naomi from IT." Naomi from IT is my "average yoga teacher" muse, who inspires my teaching of yoga teachers. In my mind, Naomi is a parent in her forties who works a desk job, and she did her yoga teacher training with her local studio. She offers "Mindful Movement" sessions at her workplace on Thursdays, and is planning on teaching a bit more when she retires. Naomi inspires my guidance in this book—as a yoga teacher, you may find creating an image of the "average practitioner" can help provide insights that are adaptable to the places and people of your community.

Even if you have an "advanced" yoga posture practice, if you teach yoga, it is unlikely your students will only be equally elite movers. Learning to teach who shows up is an act of creativity and compassion.

When Mick Jagger and The Rolling Stones first started playing together, they were developing their style in tiny venues, with even tinier stages. Their equipment took up so much space that Jagger developed his signature dance style by accomplishing what movements he could within the constraints of a small area.[4] What we perceive as limitations could be the challenges we need to hone and strengthen our methods—challenges feed creativity.

Your students will inspire your creativity. If a student comes to your class who has sciatic pain, is pregnant, has an interest in different styles of meditation, etc., you will learn to develop and expand your yoga teaching toolkit to meet the needs of your community. Your teaching will respond to the times as well as your students' goals and requirements.

In Buddhist teachings, compassion is referred to as a "quiver of the heart" in response to others' suffering. Compassion is an awareness of both our own and others' vulnerability, as well as a way of being in the world that mutually considers our inner lives. Compassion is kind connection, and there is so much satisfaction in creating inclusive, accessible yoga spaces for connection with others.

When I started teaching yoga, I initially taught classes that reflected my own movement abilities by that time—my classes required strength, and involved fluid and tricky movements. What I quickly came to realize was that my classes were exclusive. When you teach exclusive classes, if one person shows up without the necessary familiarity and abilities, what are your options? Many teachers will choose not to accommodate this student, typically because they feel pressure to deliver a class that meets the other students' expectations. Perhaps such teachers haven't learned yet that accessible, inclusive yoga doesn't have to sacrifice efficiency and strengthening.

Yoga is about union, so I couldn't ignore those students. I had to develop methods that met more people's needs. This book offers you those methods to help you approach your classes with creativity and compassion, and to inspire confidence in your students' resilience.

While it may sound like I began yoga for myself and I teach for others, the truth is that practice has a positive effect on both individuals and communities. I became a happier, more skillful person through yoga practice, which in turn made me a better family member, partner, and mother. My practice also helps me to be a better teacher.

Whatever you are teaching, there is guidance here for you. This book is a journey of collaborative discovery—I focus on methods, rather than prescriptive content. Take what is helpful to you and be a scientist of yoga—test, observe, and retest. My techniques have been refined throughout my journey, and I hope they continue to sharpen and improve, as yoga is a path of refinement.

Using This Book

This book has more information than it does pictures, because most of us have access to the internet, which can do a better job of presenting visual information than I can in this book.

Instead, I prefer to offer examples of activities and sequences you can incorporate to illustrate a point.

I believe that by learning *why* you do something, you will develop into an innovator of practice through your discovery and experimentation. I also encourage you to take workshops with the many excellent movement educators out there in your community. In essence, every movement and yoga style has something to offer, and movement is best explored through in-person instruction.

Many sections have "journaling activities" to help inspire your thinking and practical application. These activities are an invitation to develop and reflect on your perspectives and adapt the content of your classes to meet the needs of your community. If you are a yoga teacher trainer, these sections could be homework for your trainees.

This book covers a broad swath of topics relevant to the teaching of yoga. As you will likely discover on your journey, there are so many fields of inquiry that are relevant to yoga. I have tried to provide a foundational introduction to many of the core concepts, and you can decide where to deepen your study.

The tradition of Mahayana Buddhism includes the bodhisattva vows, which include the maxim "None of us are there until we are all there." The bodhisattva is an almost-awakened being who postpones their own enlightenment in order to help other beings reach the same place. What a lofty, impossible goal! However, we set lofty, impossible goals to compel us toward trying with enthusiasm. The learning of all things relevant to yoga is such a big goal, but we set it to remind ourselves that there is so much more to study, and we will always be learning.

It is very possible that you will have to come back to this book a few times. There are a lot of suggestions for refining your teaching practice, and change happens in stages. You will need to adopt a few recommendations and test them, observe the results, and test them again. You will need to practice, and can always return to the book for other methods as your skills and opportunities for refinement evolve.

Further, the vastness of yoga is such that we will never know it all. Some of the ideas may seem too challenging or not suitable for you *today*, but they may be suitable in the future, after you've done some more teaching and learning. My favorite yoga books are the ones I feel always have more to offer me as my teaching practice develops and evolves over the years, and I hope this book will live on your shelf for reading now, and for reading in the future.

A Brief History of Yoga's Definition

Defining yoga can be simple in some ways, while also remaining immensely complex and hotly contested. Once they feel initiated, many yogis vigorously police the boundaries of yoga, while others feel more generous and just declare that "everything is yoga." For these reasons, I think every book on yoga has a section with this same title.

As one of my teachers, Michael Stone, said, "There is no yoga without your life." Yoga, like any philosophy, evolves to meet the needs of the era.

While I think that every moment of your life offers opportunities for spiritual and ethical practice, considering what constitutes yoga honors your relationship to yoga. Relationships where one side always gives and the other always takes are unsustainable; for a balanced relationship with yoga, we have to accept responsibility for how we practice shaping yoga as a whole.

We must ask ourselves: *What elements of yoga do I want to survive? How, as a yoga teacher, am I more responsible for its survival than the people who take my classes?*

This may lead us toward thinking about the commodification of yoga—when yoga becomes just another sphere for driving consumerism (I've seen yoga sell everything from insurance, to yogurt). Our behavior shapes culture, including consumer culture, which means we can be a part of positive cultural shifts by examining our behavior.

Of course, that doesn't mean we need to punish or exclude others for engaging with yoga in ways that do good in their lives but are "only" physical, or that involve trendy elements, like adding in goats! If the barrier of entry to yoga only admitted those of the highest moral and spiritual order, many of us would not be sitting here—myself included. If we want to teach yoga, however, we must consider the political and ethical impact that our efforts have on our communities and the broader yoga community as a whole.

In North America, yoga has a reputation as a group exercise activity involving a lot of systematic stretching and strengthening postures. As our relationship to yoga matures, we come to appreciate that these classes are *"yoga-asana,"* making up one element of a multifaceted system of philosophy and spirituality.

You are likely aware that the word "yoga" means "union," since the Sanskrit word can translate as "to yoke." This definition stems from the group of texts called the *Vedas*—the wisdom, or knowledge—which were set down between 1,500 and 1,000 BCE. The yoking referred to here was that of a horse to a chariot; in its evolution, it became the union of body and mind.

On the way, yoga had many, many, *many* meanings. If you look at Sir William Monier's definitive Sanskrit-to-English dictionary, the definition of yoga is too long to reasonably include in this book, since it takes up over four columns of print and has 2,500 attributed words. Some of my favorite definitions include *deceit, expedient device, magic trick, business,* and *suitably fit,* in part because I find that "expedient device" is a great definition of yoga. I also find so much joy in sharing these unexpected translations with yoga teacher trainees, who believe that yoga is magical, but not a magic trick.

Developing from the yoking of chariots and horses, the definition of "yoga" began to include the warrior in the chariot. The chariot is the warrior's "expedient device," allowing him to skillfully travel on his path (and it would have definitely been a "him" in those days). The word "yoga" emerged before the practice of yoga did—it was a common word at least until around 1,200 BCE, by which point it had come to mean a discipline to control the mind and senses, a definition that remains relatively unchanged since then.

The warrior definition may be surprising, but yoga's source texts are replete with war and warrior imagery. *Yoga-asana* has its Warrior postures, and often evokes tools of war, such as bows and arrows. This imagery makes more sense when you contextualize yogic study with the *Bhagavad Gita* (the Song of the Lord) and histories of the place now called India.

Up here in Canada, we may think we're doing pretty well at welcoming diversity. However, India is truly a place of incredible diversity—they have 22 officially recognized languages today, and over 1,500 mother tongues by other counts. This cradle of civilization has such a diversity of faiths and philosophies, and within each, there are different schools of thought. Like the rest of the world, India's history includes groups of people pitted against one another to secure land and power. We may think of yogis as peaceful beings, outside the political movements of society (the "hippies" of every era), and yes, yoga's history features many ascetics purposefully living outside society. However, yoga has been wielded in different ways in each era—history has even seen roving bands of yogis control city-states,[5] not unlike gangs of the modern era.

The history of yoga is immense. If I were to ask you to summarize what's happened in English literature in the last 100 years, it would be a daunting task, if not an impossible one. Given yoga's longevity and the number of cultures, languages, religions, and philosophies yoga has touched, it is wise to anchor your study in a specific text or school. If the earlier history of yoga interests you, I highly recommend David Gordon White's *Yoga Sutras: A Biography*, which uses Patanjali's *Yoga Sutras* to lead you from yoga's earlier history to the shores of North America.

To study yoga without losing our minds to the frustration of enormous history, we must acknowledge that cultural evolution is not linear and tidy. Yoga, like all ideas, spread to various places through the people that practiced and taught it, and since all communities rise and fall, so too do ideas and trends. Some yoga even circulated back into Indic culture to evolve itself after heading elsewhere and returning. Yoga developed in multiple countries and influenced various religions, including Hinduism, Buddhism, and Jainism.[6]

While many perceive yoga as merely an effective stretching regimen, try not to be discouraged by other people's ideas about your practice. In the same way that you may attend a bake sale at a school or church that you have no affiliation with, some people attend services, and other people try to lead them. There are both casual and committed ways of engaging any practice. In fact, by the second century of the Common Era, yoga was sufficiently established such that many laypeople practiced elements of yoga as a regular part of their lives, and others adopted it exclusively as a lifestyle and became renunciates (*sannyasins*) who lived outside society. Yoga has a long history of people using it for different reasons.

Practically speaking, yoga is a pragmatic program. When I say this in social conversations, I am often met with some skepticism. To me, nothing could be more practical. Yoga and its sister science, Ayurveda, are tools of intervention: *Are you feeling a certain way and would like to change that? Here is how you go about that.* These systems are replete with tools for reorienting our behavior toward clarity and healthfulness.

Taking care of the body with exercise (*yoga-asana*) and breathwork (*pranayama*) helps us feel good in our bodies and minds. Learning to discipline the mind through meditation (*dhyana*) helps us diminish the power of harmful mental patterns and align ourselves with more helpful patterns. The system moves from addressing the more obvious needs of physical manifestation (i.e., having a body) toward the more subtle needs of having a spirit, but the two are not separate. What feels magical about yoga is that these practices both address the real needs of bodies and minds, such as reducing lower back pain or stress, *and* produce spiritual experiences.

The "union" of yoga evolved to become the interconnectedness of all beings, and we can feel a sense of unity with the universe beyond our separate selves. Historical yogis discerned that natural laws govern the material world, and they are discernable to increasingly fine degrees. That is one of the things I love about teaching yoga—you are not teaching people secrets of magic that they can access only through you and by your methods, you are teaching them tools of awareness that allow them to experience insight firsthand.

That might sound grand, but yoga's spirituality is also quite pragmatic—you do not need to pray and conduct rituals with your fingers crossed, hoping that a deity issues decisions in your favor. Like Buddhism, these systems can be viewed as practical programs that empower the practitioner to test the tools for themselves and observe the reactions to their actions. The teachings orient us toward our true identity as a spiritual being, whether it is called the aware self (*atman*), or spirit (*purusha*).

Yoga, like other spiritual paths, helps us "wake up" in our lives. It allows us to see where we are suffering needlessly, and how we can navigate unavoidable pain and discomfort in a more skillful way. We call yoga a science because the outcomes of practice are predictable. Through the practices of yoga, if you engage with the right intentions, you can break free of habitual patterns of thinking (*samskaras*), particularly your over-identification with your body/mind.

As I discuss throughout the book, my methods change with testing, observation, and responding to the needs of my current students. The yoga that you teach may occasionally feel repetitive, but let me reassure you that yoga endures because of its predictable outcomes. The flavor and perspective you bring to yoga may feel like a creative, artistic endeavor, but as a yoga teacher, you are part of a long history of yoga scientists.

PART ONE

Bringing Philosophy and Ethics to Life

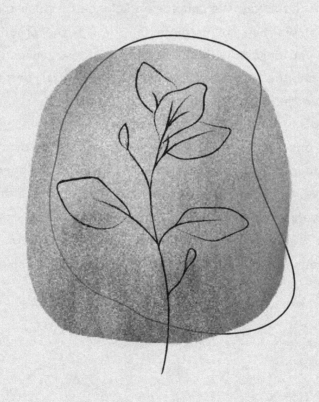

YOGA SHARES A COMMON history with Hinduism in that it is born of the *Vedas*, a set of some of the oldest religious texts known to humankind. *Veda* is Sanskrit for "wisdom," and so yoga and its sister science, Ayurveda, are called Vedic sciences: sciences of wisdom.

Ayurveda is often translated as "the wisdom of life," but a more active translation is "living wisdom." We generate wisdom by applying our knowledge from study to how we live; observing the outcome and orienting future behavior forms our wisdom. Yoga philosophy provides a foundation of knowledge for this reason.

It's important to note that if you have a preexisting religion or philosophy, there is no need to pick one or the other. As we explore in the upcoming section on cultural appropriation, bringing yoga into all elements of your life is part of responsible use. Yoga does not have a discrete history anyway; philosophies evolve through the places and people who touch them.

The *Vedas* beg the question that all philosophies and religions arose to answer in the ancient world: What are we doing here? Without the scientific knowledge of evolution and earth's history, simply existing can be confusing. All creation myths address the fundamental predicament of existence, our wondering of questions like *How did we get here, and what does it all mean?*

While we may know a lot more about the material world now, the question "What are we doing here?" is a good place to begin thinking about your yoga practice and your teaching practice. Why do you want to teach yoga? What do you hope to gain from it?

Once creation myths are established, it's time to improve life upon this earth (*prakriti*). Religions and philosophies are shaped to meet the needs of the day, and while the causes of suffering change over the millennia and various geographies, yoga arises as a solution to suffering for some of our enduring needs. Those needs include mastery over the self and guidance on moral living.

The philosophies and faiths of the India peninsula often believed in rebirth: you were born, lived, died, and were reborn. Your rebirth reflected the caliber of your actions (*karma*) in your previous life. The very nature of the material realm (*prakriti*) is cyclical—everything comes into existence, exists for a time, and then dissolves.

The seers, or *rishis*, of Ayurveda, like the yogis and Buddhists, saw a cyclical pattern to nature reflected in the seasons, as well as the life cycle. They determined that these cycles of nature influenced us because we are made of nature, made of the same elements, thus, we are subject to material impermanence and influenced by the natural world.

There are simple examples to illustrate this wisdom. If we are outside during a spring rain, we will feel wet and cold because water is wet and cold. To feel dry, we balance the wetness of rain by wearing protective clothing, and banish the cold by finding a heat source. If we are feeling cold of heart, we can practice heartwarming *mantras* (a sacred utterance that focuses the mind and aligns intentions) to connect us with feelings of compassion, and we can perform active movements that produce endorphins (chemical messengers of the nervous system), which will warm up our heart.

Beyond nature we are spirit. The spirit that resides in us, our consciousness, is a reminder that we are actually drops of divine essence having an embodied experience. Put simply, we are not just live bodies; we are spiritual beings with bodies! When we forget that we are spiritual beings, born of a universal consciousness, we overly identify with the little cruelties and possessions of the material realm. We become egocentric— life may feel like only bad things are happening to us, and we may be less charitable toward others. We are not practicing the "union" of our yoga; instead, we are clinging to the idea of separateness. As yoga teachers, that may look like rejecting feedback on our teaching without due consideration, or feeling jealous of the perceived success of another teacher.

If you're clear on why you're teaching yoga and develop a practice/lifestyle rooted in compassion, you will be able to steer yourself away from participating in those less-healthful attachments.

Personal Change:
The Yoga Sutras

Yoga Has Limits

THIS BOOK BEGINS WITH some of yoga's history, including the philosophical texts describing how to cultivate personal and community change. While I wouldn't write a book about yoga without believing in its profound ability to promote wellness, it's important to remember that yoga has limits. Where yoga and Western self-improvement culture meet, the practice can become conflated, becoming a tool to make ourselves more acceptable, rather than a journey of learning to accept ourselves.

When you teach yoga, you offer a forum for self-observation. Students learn to look within and ask, *How do I feel today? What is happening in my inner world?* Their yoga practice affirms for them the medicine of contemplative practices, exercise, and time away from screens. Sometimes there is a straight line to be drawn between behavior and effects. As we grow more sensitive to the impact of our actions, our practice becomes ever more responsive to the subtle consequences our actions have on our bodies and minds. We start to make connections about our wellness that aren't quite as obvious.

While this book examines techniques for personal and professional refinement, it's important to also state that some things in your life are not yours to fix or to work on alone. Sometimes what needs to change is our relationship to a thought, or to a person. No amount of yoga practice can make an abusive relationship right, and excessive rumination on negative thoughts that plague us requires more support than yoga alone can provide. Other paths to achieving peace and mental wellness include therapy and social worker support.

Even though evidence that yoga practices are beneficial for both physical and behavioral health continues to mount, some of our expectations of yoga can be unrealistic, and may feed harmful interpretations about ideal embodiment.

We know that culture prescribes these ideals—certain bodies, ages, and faces dominate advertising and media (even yoga media), and we internalize these ideals through constant exposure. We may not explicitly set the goal of aligning with those ideals, but these pressures reveal themselves in other ways.

For example, if you get an injury, become ill, or have a significant life change, you may not be able to practice as frequently, or in the same way. In addition to potentially feeling less comfortable in our bodies if we aren't practicing, some dark thoughts may come up too. We may think that without our physical practice, we will fall short.

In your classes, please be sensitive to where you may be promoting these harmful ideas. An example would be saying things like "We're doing this core sequence so we can earn our Thanksgiving dinner!" Comments like this perpetuate the idea that yoga should produce a look (external), rather than allowing us to process our experiences (internal).

As yoga teachers, we offer practices that can help students meet life's challenges, but not prevent or cure them. Keeping in mind that yoga is just one tool of many, that yoga can be used for helpful and harmful purposes, and that some needs exceed yoga's scope, let's look at some of the texts for guidance on personal and community change.

As part of your yoga teacher training, you may have read the *Yoga Sutras* or the *Bhagavad Gita*. These popular yoga texts are two of many, but together they offer a path to thinking about our personal practice of yoga and our practice in community. Since familiarity with the history of these yogic texts is essential for any yoga teacher, and commitment to philosophy varies in terms of training, I believe it is important to offer you some background.

The Myth of Patanjali

The sage Patanjali set down the *Yoga Sutras* a few hundred years before the Common Era, but it's maybe more accurate to say "Patanjalis." It's possible that multiple authors accredited their work to this one teacher, which is hard to believe in an era where trademarked yoga "methods" are abundant. Sometimes titles derive from family names, so the Flynn Sutra could have been written by my whole family.

We don't know much about Patanjali, but he does have his own creation myth. He was a sage who came to the earth after Lord Vishnu heard many prayers for help coping with the diseases of body, mind, and speech. Vishnu sent the sacred serpent, Adi Shesha, to appear in material form on Earth and write the treatise that would offer cures.

For that incarnation to take place, he had to be born. A yogini named Gonika was praying to Surya the Sun God for a son, and as she prayed, a child with a snake's tail (or a tiny snake, depending on the version of the story and its translation) fell into her open palms. Her prayers were answered, and she had a child to whom she could pass on her yogic wisdom.

Like many Sanskrit words, Patanjali is a compound word. *Pata* means "to fall," and *anjali* means "hands" or "prayer"—you may recognize *anjali* from the connected-palms *mudra* used to close yoga classes.

The Text

On a macro level, the *Yoga Sutras* are a set of instructions for overcoming the cyclical turning of embodiment (incarnation over and over again) and achieving *moksha*, freedom. If we achieve awareness of the indivisibility of all beings, we will no longer be reincarnated, forced to struggle through life on earth.

Breaking free from cyclical suffering is desirable. I mentioned earlier that philosophies and religions arise and evolve to meet the needs of the day, and those needs almost always include guidance on the unfairness of life. Why do some people have so much opportunity and privilege when others have so little? The *Yoga Sutras* offer less reflection on this question than the *Gita* does, but they do offer guidance for the individual seeking to change their circumstances.

On the micro level, yoga provides the techniques (or technology) to free ourselves from the cyclical nature of suffering and live with more ease. The text of the *Yoga Sutras* presents a technology of the self; a recipe for personal transformation that was intended for individuals who renounced householder life and became ascetic yogis.

As lofty as that sounds, Patanjali is not poetic in his technical direction. The *Sutras* themselves are pithy and to the point. There are only four verbs in the entire collection, and since verbs are action words that give direction, reading the *Sutras* is a lifetime process of discussion and study. Good quality commentary from academics and discussion on how the text relates to modern practice makes its wisdom meaningful in our lives.

The *Yoga Sutras* synthesize many ideas or schools of thought into one compendium, so there is repetition within it—though I have no doubt the adherents to those various discrete threads of yoga would argue they are not substitutions for one another. When you read the *Sutras*, you'll find that what Patanjali just said in one way seems a lot like what he said another way. Your perception is correct!

The most popular extraction from the *Yoga Sutras* is the eight-limb path of yoga (*ashtanga*), a prescription of yogic ethics, practices, and outcome. The limbs are restraints (*yama*), observances (*niyama*), postures (*asana*), breath control (*pranayama*), sensory withdrawal (*pratyahara*), fixed meditation (*dharana*), abstract meditation (*dhyana*), and absorption (*samadhi*).

The *Sutras*' eight-limb path has become the definitive path in modern Western yoga culture, but the history to its popularity is fascinating (involving a too-often-forgotten historical figure known as "Madame Blavatsky"), and it's not the only multi-limb path out there. There are other yogic texts with different limbs to the yogic path. Sometimes the limbs are mostly similar—the *Gheranda Samhita* has seven limbs, and the *Goraksha Samhita* has six. Within the *Yoga Sutras*, Patanjali also sets forth a three-limb path, if you will, consisting of discipline (*tapas*), self-study and/or study of scriptures (*svadhyaya*), and devotion to the Lord, or divine (*isvara pranidhana*).

There is no singular yoga lineage, no vertical progression of yoga. What becomes popular has to do with who championed which text at which time, and is subject to the whims of history. While there are certainly teachings that have been preserved and passed on, there is murkiness to the history of yoga, since it is so vast and enduring.

Habits and Mindfulness

Yoga philosophy has abundant advice on what we call "habits," and what Patanjali conceptualizes as "*samskaras*." *Samskaras* are mental formations that build up over years of thinking and acting. In Patanjali's *Yoga Sutras*, they translate into English as "latent impressions," because, like all habits, they are subtle at first and take form only after repetition. I think of them as "grooves of the mind," evoking the brain's grooved appearance.

Have you ever stood on a sand bar in the ocean, feeling the snaking ridges of soft sand under your feet? The surface of the ocean may be still, but the currents beneath continue to imprint upon the sand below. Often, we are not consciously trying to form these grooves of our mind, but they appear nonetheless, because our minds are constantly moving and interpreting our outer experiences.

A strong component of habits is that they are often unconscious actions, and most undesirable habits develop unintentionally.[7] No one intends to stay up late, scrolling on their phone—it's the unintentional behavior that forms the habit. Cultivating self-awareness, which yoga helps us achieve, allows us to be more intentional with how we spend our energy.

Yoga draws attention to our thoughts and our words. Think of how many times you've realized during class that you were somewhere else entirely—writing an email, rehashing a conversation, or planning another part of your day. The invitation of yoga is to be with the present moment and watch it unfold without applying personal coloring, interpretation, or reaction.

Through mindfulness, we illuminate our unconsciously patterned harmful or limiting *samskaras* and purposefully repattern them. The techniques of *yoga-asana—pranayama*, meditation, *mantra*, etc.—are the tools we use for practice. Our practices help us live more deliberately, releasing us from harmful patterns and maintaining or nurturing desirable ones.

Since these patterns are often unconscious, to decondition the mind and be more intentional in our behavior is a way of "waking up" in our lives. Patanjali says that witnessing these latent impressions (*samskaras*) perfectly gives us great insight—so powerful that we'll know about our previous incarnations!

Yes, Patanjali promises magical powers (including levitation!), which was common to philosophies of the time; even Buddhism has a history of magic. Patanjali says that knowing ourselves reveals our past and forthcoming incarnations, and they represent a cycle of cause and effect, or action and outcome. Cultivating self-awareness illuminates our personal cycles of action and outcome, giving us the opportunity to refine our actions (*karma*).

You have likely noticed that your mind is a more peaceful place to be after a yoga class, some exercise, or time in nature. We know that taking care of our physical body is an essential part of developing a healthy mind, but increasing our awareness of the movements of our minds and reducing our reactivity is a part of repatterning too.

The common term is mindfulness: the moment-to-moment awareness of what is happening right now. That definition may seem obvious, but think about the practice of *Savasana* for a moment. We often try to dress it up as a magical experience (though I am not condemning the magic of being left alone to breathe with yourself for 10 minutes). Still, *Savasana* is, essentially, lying on the floor on a rectangular piece of rubber and being aware that you have a body that is breathing. The imaginary realms in your mind can make the moment quite fantastical—you can be in so many other places, having so many different conversations—but here you are in this humble space. You are lying on the floor, on a rectangular piece of rubber, being aware of your breathing. Mindfulness is the awareness that the realms are not real, and you are here, on the floor, in order to experience what is real: the present moment of air moving into your body and moving out. Inhaling, and exhaling.

Mindfulness practices are intervention techniques for shortening the distance between being in those imaginary realms and the real present moment. Minds are always going to wander, but your mastery over returning to the present moment improves. Beyond meditation, we can employ *mantra*, journaling, conscious breathing, and, of course, mindful movement throughout our days. Where there is mindfulness, there is less risk of swerving into the grooves we are trying to repattern.

Journaling Activity

Has teaching yoga become another internal distraction in your practices? How can you create some distinction between your teaching planning and your personal practice?

Your Elemental Makeup

In case our yoga exploration so far has a "one size fits all" flavor to it, before we continue, let's embrace the idea that we can each have a unique relationship with yoga. There is no ideal yoga practice, and that will be self-evident if you also embrace yoga's sister system, Ayurveda ("living wisdom").

I describe the relationship between yoga and Ayurveda this way: If yoga is a system of practices helping your integrated body and mind (bodymind) break free from limiting behaviors and beliefs, your bodymind needs to be cared for using a lifestyle and medicinal system that supports those practices. Since it makes sense to us that healing practices are applied based on our unique needs, it helps us see that yoga's practices must be individually tailored, too.

There are many resources available to you to help you study Ayurveda, a lifestyle that emphasizes wellness and the prevention of disease. However, there is an essential pillar of Ayurveda I want to highlight for our compassionate yoga lens.

You may have heard of Ayurveda's idea of *dosha*, typically translated as "composition" or "constitution," to describe why people differ physically and psychologically. Fun fact: it actually means "blemish", "default," or "mistake," since it's the nature of nature to be constantly changing, giving us new situations to adjust to—providing opportunities to further tailor our behavior.

The concept of *dosha* stems from the understanding that nature has five elements of structure: space/ether (*akasha*), air/wind (*vayu*), fire (*agni*), water (*jala*), and earth (*prthvi*). Since we are a part of nature, we are also composed of these five elements. Everyone has all five elements (no matter what your five-minute internet quiz tells you about your fire), and each element has qualities (*gunas*) that influence how we experience embodiment.

For example, we all have fire as a part of our makeup. That fire manifests both physiologically and psychologically, as it allows us to digest food and process incoming information. Some people have more fire than others, so their digestion may be faster. People with fast digestion and lots of fire in their constitution will want to be mindful that they do not stoke their fire too much, because that could result in speeding up the process of elimination too much. There are many yogic practices that stoke our internal fire, so it follows that we apply them only when there's a need to harness the fire element.

The idea is that, even though everyone has the same elemental building blocks, they manifest in different ways and appear in varying quantities. We are each uniquely affected by the elements when seasons change and when seasons of life change. Studying Ayurveda gives us the gift of understanding that what is an appropriate practice for one person at one time is not the proper practice for someone else (I hope this helps explain why your friend loves hot yoga and you just don't get it).

The study of Ayurveda also provides a reminder that different approaches to practice all have a place in our yoga toolkit—what determines their success is skillful, timely application.

Individuality is the Theme: Ayurveda and Neurodiversity

Even though we can cultivate change, there is another term to introduce to our compassionate yoga lens: *neurodiversity.*

Neurodiversity first emerged as a term used to describe people on the autism spectrum, as well as people with dyslexia, social anxiety disorders, ADHD, and so on. It expresses that the bodymind embodiment in these cases is a variation of a theme, and not a corruption of normalcy.

In music composition, different sections of a musical work can be radically different, totally unrecognizable as parts of a whole. A *leitmotif* is a unifying theme; an element that appears throughout, reminding the listener of the "wholeness" of the overall piece. A leitmotif could be a particular use of a decorative note, a short melody, etc. How does this apply to yoga? Well, we have already talked about the *Yoga Sutras* (threads of yoga), and you may have realized that the Sanskrit word *sutra* (thread) shares a root with suture. Like a suture, a leitmotif stitches things together.

Human embodiment works the same way: We are each a variation on a theme, yet we all possess elements that unite us. While our vocal cords are all basically built the same way, slight variations in their formation produce different voices.

That is why you may sound a lot like one of your parents or siblings, but you cannot sound *exactly* the same— as you age, your tissues change, and thus your voice changes.

Yoga teachers understand that, like the variety of bodies that you might have in one class, people come to practice with different minds and experiences. This means that, in the same way we are increasingly sensitive to how people physically experience a class, we can invite that same open-endedness to how people mentally experience a class. What is grounding for one person may be aggravating for another; what one person finds challenging might be easy for someone else.

The aim is not to have a class that perfectly meets the needs of a diverse group of people, but to cultivate invitations to explore our unique experiences in a group setting.

Change in Community: The Bhagavad Gita

EARLIER IN THE BOOK, I mentioned your personal relationship to yoga, which we will see takes various forms. One of the strangest social aspects about teaching yoga classes is that you often talk *at* people, rather than *with* them. The conversation loop is rarely closed, unless you have one of those rare, delightful students who shout questions in the middle of class (I hear you, Brian!). Yoga teachers often connect and talk to each other more on social media than they do in person, especially if you're mostly teaching in a workplace or other setting where yoga is not the main focus.

As much as yoga is a technology of self-development, this is not a book on how to be an ascetic, someone who renounces society to demonstrably live outside it. Like me, you are probably a *grastha*, or "householder," someone who is going to have a place to live, a family, a job, etc. Living your yoga is about your relationship to self, as we discussed in the previous section, but also your relationship to others in various circles of your community.

When we come to a practice, we filter that practice through the lens of our reality—the names and ideas that are relevant to us. We want to make our lives easier, and that is a fine, even good, thing to do.

However, how we use something influences what it becomes—I say this all the time when I teach "Pigeon pose" *(Kapotasana)*. The floppy, one-legged Pigeon bum stretch (*Eka Pada Kapotasana)* most people associate with the word "pigeon" used to be an upright backbend in preparation for an enormous backbend, *Kapotasana*, or Pigeon pose. Look it up! It's an insane backbend!

Everyone kept calling the bum stretch pose "pigeon," and as time passed, that's what it became. I don't think there's a real loss here to investigate, but I want to emphasize that small, consistent efforts can make cultural changes. How we use something is what it becomes; how we use yoga shapes it, and how we are in our community shapes that community. Uniting our intentions and actions is a part of yoga practice, and an aspect that we can carry into relationships. That's why we may need some advice; fortunately, yoga philosophy has some to give.

Patanjali's *Yoga Sutras*, and later medieval-era texts like the *Hatha Yoga Pradipika*, offer instructions for personal transformation. The *Bhagavad Gita* explores how we can participate yogically in a community. Techniques take us inward, and ethical inquiry guides our outward behavior. This balance of inward reflection to inform outward ethical action reminds me of one of my favorite Sanskrit words, *spanda*, which literally means "pulsation" or "vibration." It refers to the expanding and contracting movement of the universe, but yoga philosophy describes your mind's movement as a reflection of the universe's qualities (*gunas*).

As I mentioned earlier, we should be particularly curious about the ethical component of yogic living if we, as teachers, are standard bearers of yoga. When yogis think of ethics, we may begin with "the *yamas* and *niyamas*" of Patanjali, but the weightiest concept of cause and effect is that of *karma*.

The word *karma* derives from the root *kri*, meaning "to make or do," and classically it means "cause and effect from lifetime to lifetime." *Karma* includes intentions, actions, and their effects. *Karma* is central to the *Gita*'s story, explored through a conversation between Prince Arjuna and Krishna, an *avatar* (embodiment) of the Hindu God, Vishnu.

The verses of the *Gita* are typically chanted, hence its title of *The Song of the Lord*. The story centers on the struggles of Prince Arjuna, who is stuck in the middle of a war between factions of his family. Studying the story as a metaphor, it prompts the question: What battle are you facing in your life right now? It's an invitation to think about how we can meet our personal needs while also meeting the needs of our community.

Prince Arjuna's dilemma is this: A cousin, Duryodhana, and his brothers have claimed Arjuna's brother's throne. He can participate in this war on behalf of his side of the family, or abandon his duty, both as a warrior and as a loyal brother. Torn between killing his kinsmen and fulfilling his familial duties,

Arjuna sinks into depression. In his depression, he asks for guidance from Krishna.

Krishna gives Arjuna a first-rate education on everything from the nature of reality to what it means to uphold your obligations and purpose, or *dharma*. While Arjuna weighs the negative consequences of action or inaction, Krishna reminds him that neither are without their *karma*—sometimes *not* participating is more harmful than participating in the world.

When we learn the word *dharma*, we may have ideas about our work, but *dharma* is much more than just our work. The term *dharma* derives from the Sanskrit root *dhr*, meaning to "hold or carry." My teacher, Mona Warner, has a wonderful way of expressing your *dharma* as upholding "your little corner of the universe." Your *dharma* encompasses your obligations to your family, friends, and community. What responsibilities fall under that umbrella and how you uphold them forms your ethical inquiry.

Yes, some people will see their work and the structure of their family as a significant part of their *dharma*, and indeed, they are both significant contributors to the shape of your life. If you were to write down all the ways in which you view yourself—as a yogi, sister, friend, Canadian, neighbor, member of humanity, etc.—you could consider how your daily life is upholding the *dharma* of these relationships. Of course, the push and pull of these obligations often forms the inspiration for yoga practice. Many people need space to cultivate self-compassion because they feel they're underperforming in one role, or many.

The important question you must ask yourself is, *What battle are you facing in your life right now?* That battle may present itself as the oppressive feeling of "too much *dharma*"; evidence that there may be insufficient or misapplied practice and support in your life. Your yoga classes will offer students a place to digest the busy-ness of their lives and find some clarity about how to be in their lives skillfully. As yoga teachers, it's imperative we have clearly defined practice in our lives.

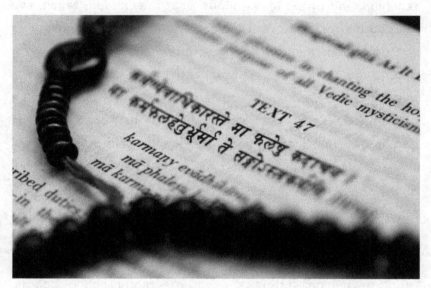

The Bhagavad Gita is written in slokas (verses) and is meant to be sung. This is verse 2.47, a popular verse describing effort and non-attachment.

In verses 2.47 and 2.50 of the *Gita*, Krishna famously says that yoga is "perfect evenness of mind" and "skill in action," which both describe a yogi who is confidently established in their sense of self. This does not mean that we learn to cope with every little thing on our plate, rather that we must constantly reassess where we are taking on someone else's *dharma*. We have a responsibility to others, yes, but sometimes we overreach and take on more than our own share. As the *Gita* concludes, in verse 18.47, it is "better to perform one's own *dharma* imperfectly than to master the duties of another."

I think of this whenever my son, Harvey, is learning a new skill and I have to think about the right amount of help to offer. I think of it when students ask for advice on their own teaching, and I have ideas about what they should teach. I've learned many times over that it's my *dharma* to ask questions and offer guidance, but not prescriptions.

Dharma can include many aspects of this life. One person's *dharma* may be tending their beautiful garden, which is itself a contemplative practice. Gardening meets their needs, and the garden becomes a sight of beauty for their community.

Some activities, like gardening, are a pleasant way to think about *dharma*, but our *dharma* also includes our larger communities and the responsibilities we have to each other. What are the forces that shape our lives? They include the way we structure communities (at a variety of levels, such as incorporating townships, setting up governments and school boards, and delineating countries), as well as the culture we shape through our behavior. The ways we vote, volunteer, and participate in shaping our world are a part of our *dharma*.

However, our *dharma* is much more than what we do—it's also *how* we are in the world.

Krishna says to Arjuna in 4.18-19,

> *The wise see that there is action in the midst of inaction and inaction in the midst of action. Their consciousness is unified, and every act is done with complete awareness. The awakened sages call a person wise when all his undertakings are free from anxiety about results; all his selfish desires have been consumed in the fire of knowledge.*

The universe is always progressing, a vibrating energy in constant motion (*spanda*). Stillness, silence, and absence exist in your perception, and introverted practice invites us to attune to ever more subtle movements and actions around us. The skillful action we perform should be *sattvic*, a blissful, peaceful state of mind. Krishna tells Arjuna in 17.15 that someone who is *sattvic* would "offer soothing words, to speak truly, kindly, and helpfully." Our yoga can be socially engaged—using active participation in shaping community—but that engagement should reflect the potency of yogic practice.

I'm not at all saying there is no place for difficult feelings or anger in yogic life; instead, I'm pointing out that we often approach engagement in community readied for battle. We go into life steeled against other perspectives and with a competitive spirit. Engaging with others forms a practice of effort (*abhyasa*) and letting go (*vairagya*), which you may recognize as a teaching from Patanjali in sutra 1.12. As Krishna says in 3.21, "What the outstanding person does, others will try to do. The standards such people create will be followed by the world."

If we are so committed to yoga that we call ourselves teachers, our skillful way of being in the world is all the promotion yoga needs.

Journaling Activity

• •

List some of your favorite yoga practices from past and present. Write down the effects that specific practices have for you, such as grounding, anxiety-reducing, confidence-building, etc. Then write down the specific ways you see yourself showing up differently in your life when your practice is meeting your needs—it could be "more patient with my kids," "better at being realistic with my to-do list," and/or "less cranky because my knees bother me less."

Connecting the lines between cause and effect on ever more subtle levels constitutes the practice of yoga. Consider this activity again and again in the future to remind yourself of benchmarks of progress.

Diversity in Yoga

When it comes to Sharing Privilege, the driving question is:

"What would be possible if we treated each other, and ourselves, as though we were important, sacred and holding some form of trauma?"

Privilege is a thing that folks have a hard time owning. I get it; perhaps the belief is if one acknowledges they have privilege, it means denying the work, the suffering, the challenges that they had to go through. But, privilege is not something to deny or be ashamed of. The privilege you have doesn't discredit the challenges you've had to overcome. Your privilege speaks to what resources you have to share. Resources aren't just physical things or wealth. It's also time, attention and the emotional toolkit required to have difficult conversations while remaining compassionate and oriented toward mutual understanding.

Don't waste your energy denying your privilege or defending the fact that you're a good person. You're human. Humans are inherently harmful. We're a terrible species. We are equally destructive as we are creative. When you feel yourself getting defensive, take a sacred pause and breathe. Then put your energy in unpacking your unconscious biases so you cause less harm. You're harmful and a good person.

- Robin Lacambra (she/her), movement educator, creator of GOODBODYFEEL Movement Studio and the Sharing Privilege Course

Throughout yoga's history, entire populations of people were excluded from participation because of their circumstances of birth, or caste.[8] The caste system in India has ancient roots, but elements of this exclusionary social hierarchy remain present, even today. Caste discrimination has been illegal in India since 1950, but discrimination persists, particularly for the Dalits, a group of people technically outside the caste system, historically called the "Untouchables."[9] In modern Western yoga culture, exclusion is less codified, but still a powerful force shaping the landscape.

As an able-bodied, cisgender (my gender identity and sex assigned at birth correspond), middle-class white woman, there are aspects of exclusion with which I do not have experience. I will offer some encouragement instead.

In Ayurveda, we say that everything begins subtly and manifests into more tangible material from there. That's why, when we consider diversity in yoga, we have to think about both the subtle ways we perpetuate a homogenous yoga culture, and tangible ways of responding to it.

If you teach yoga, you likely believe in its benefits and feel it should be available to any interested student. However, people may be unlikely to participate in a community where the practitioners, teachers, and leaders do not look like them. When we support and promote teachers from diverse backgrounds, embodiments, and perspectives, we not only broaden our understanding of yoga and self-inquiry by hearing different perspectives, we also say to the broader community, *yoga is for you too.*

When we make an effort to use promotional images that include people of varying ages, body types, abilities, and color, we are implicitly encouraging participation from a diverse range of folks. When you choose images for your posters, handouts, and social media, consider using images of a variety of people doing yoga, or an individual who diversifies the idea that yoga is only for white, skinny, flexible young women. If you create a social media feed featuring yoga, remember that imagery conveys a powerful message. If you only post photos of yoga postures, your feed conveys that yoga is only about yoga postures—whether that is your intention or not.

A diverse student pool is ideal, but it is more achievable if we have diverse leadership. As I said earlier, learning from different perspectives that challenge our views of the world refines our understanding. That is not confrontational; one of the limitations of privilege is that we often cannot see barriers, exclusion, and prejudice because the world reflects our own lived reality. Hearing from a diversity of teachers simply reveals what we cannot see, which is a pretty "yoga" learning experience.

Diversity in leadership also offers yoga teachings to different communities in a way that is most meaningful to them. Think of a time when you needed someone who could empathize, and who understood your challenges accurately—as a parent, I know that other new parents were vital to my network of support when my son was born. While many of the teachings of yoga are universal to humanity, we need universal teachings just as much as we need teachings that speak to our own embodied experiences.

Beyond choosing yoga imagery that celebrates diversity for your promotional channels, consider taking a workshop with someone who offers a different perspective than your own. Ask your studios what they are doing to promote diversity and reduce barriers to practice, and if you decide to provide workshops and training one day, ask yourself the same question.

We should all do some self-inquiry when it comes to implicitly held beliefs about what a yoga teacher looks like. Those ideas may not show up as overtly stated principles, but they can linger as subconscious expectations that reveal themselves in our preferences and selections—who we give our attention and dollars to speaks volumes about these expectations.

Being open to exploring our capacity for being inclusive or exclusive is part of this journey toward unity (*yoga*). When I teach meditation, I talk about "the executive center" of our brain (the prefrontal cortex), and how meditation helps develop the region associated with empathy.

No matter what magic powers (*siddhis*) the yogic texts promise, meditation does not give us the ability to read other people's minds. Humans tend to like people who remind them of themselves (their favorite person!). Still, through ethical self-inquiry, yogis can increase the space in their brains used to consider other people's experiences. We can ask ourselves how we may be more inclusive, and then ask people who may be excluded about their experiences with yoga, so we can build a flourishing, more diverse yoga community.

Cultural Appropriation and Yoga

Definition

> *"Cultural appropriation is the taking, marketing, and exotification of cultural practices from historically oppressed populations. The problem is incredibly complex and involves two extremes: the first is the sterilization of yoga by removing the evidence of its Eastern roots so that it doesn't "offend" Westerner practitioners. The opposite extreme is the glamorization of yoga and India through commercialism, such as OM tattoos, T-shirts sporting Hindu deities, or Sanskrit scriptures that are often conflated with yoga, or the choosing of Indian names."*

— Rina Deshpande, yoga researcher, writer, and teacher

Tucked safely in my closet is a great treasure—a square of fabric clipped off a blanket that belonged to my grandparents. I specifically associate it with my grandfather, Harvey.

To anyone but me, it is a worthless scrap of fabric. If my husband were to use it as a dish cloth, I would reclaim it and clarify its meaning to me. Even if he doesn't share the meaning, it's a valued part of my history, and, being in relationship together, we need to respect each other's meaning-making practices. The symbols and stories of such practices are personal, spiritual, and cultural; that is, they are intensely human.

As we've touched on, yoga has a vast history of people and practices, and being a yoga teacher requires a thoughtful relationship with yoga. When we take only what we deem useful, disrespect the meaning of the practice elements, or divorce it entirely from its original context, we are participating in the cultural appropriation of yoga.

Even though yoga's history is vast, each practice leaves some trail of translations, stories, and champions. Tracing the historical trail of your practices is part of a responsible relationship to yoga. Inconsiderate use of yoga, on the other hand, is a one-sided relationship that may constitute cultural appropriation.

Cultural appropriation erases the originators of yoga and their perspectives. For some people, yoga is a cultural inheritance, but in yoga spaces that erase yoga's history, practitioners can feel like strangers in what should be a familiar land. Part of the remedy is to learn about yoga's history and the history of the people from which it came. Listen and learn from Desi voices and teachers (Desi comes from the Sanskrit *desa*, देश , and translates to country/land; it refers to the diaspora of people from the countries of India, Nepal, Bangladesh, Sri Lanka, and Pakistan).

The history and modern politics of much of yoga's iconography (symbols, deities, scripts, etc.) are more complicated than you may imagine. In contemporary Indian politics, Hindu nationalist groups and politicians sometimes use yoga to blur the lines between religious and national heritage, including the use of the OM symbol. Minorities in India sometimes feel that yoga is used to promote religious and class indoctrination. As part of your yoga practice, learn about the cultural and political context under which this practice emerges (and how it continues to be used in India) as fervently as you read the *Yoga Sutras* and the *Bhagavad Gita*.

In Practice

Ten years ago, I attended a large yoga festival and was standing in line at a food vendor. The atmosphere was pleasant, and I struck up a conversation with other attendees while we waited to inch closer toward our vegan noodle boxes. As we discussed the festival itself, I mentioned my disappointment in the festival handing out bindi stickers for folks to place on their foreheads. One woman told me that "yoga was about feeling good, and if it felt good to wear a bindi sticker, then it was yoga." I wish I had said to her that while yoga can help us feel good, it shouldn't come at the cost of someone else feeling bad (I said something way less eloquent, and it made for some quiet, awkward noodle-box waiting).

In her blog post, *How to Practice Yoga Without Appropriating It,* Susanna Barkataki writes that teaching yoga responsibly includes honoring yoga's roots, teaching and practicing all the limbs of yoga, showing a little humility and reverence through continued studentship, and embracing a spirit of uplifting each other.

She writes, "*by practicing in a heartfelt way; we do our part to bring about this golden age of people waking up to understanding their unity with one another. This unity isn't possible through ignoring difference, pretending it doesn't exist or railroading it, but only by going in, looking deeply, reflecting, and sharing with others who have a different perspective than ours."*

What are some practical guidelines? Beyond cultivating an interest and studentship of yoga's history and cultural context, here are a few practical tips.

Avoid yoga consumption. What are some of the views on how to use mala beads? Where does the practice come from? Do you use them for more than jewelry? Being able to confidently describe the history and practical uses of yoga's practice tools moves them out of superficial signaling and into a process of respectful use. Yoga is far more about how you practice and live than what yoga gear you own. Treat the objects of your practice as launch points of inquiry.

Diversify your teachers. Find voices and perspectives that are different than yours. This could include featuring teachings from South Asian and South Asian diaspora yogis. The wonder of the internet is that readings, online workshops, and classes are readily available. The most meaningful way to engage with a teacher is to support their work by enrolling in their programs, but you can also engage through conscientious participation in their social media and writing.

Question your perception. Yoga is a practice that centers on how your perception influences your action *(karma)*. How you view the world is influenced by the elements that make up your social and cultural context—your race, culture, gender, class, time in history, etc. All these factors influence how you view the world and what you deem to be useful, ethically sound, etc. It's impossible not to be influenced by these aspects of identity; it's a part of being human. However, these contexts can limit us in the ways we go about listening to others with the goal of understanding. Considering our own biases in our relationship to yoga is the other side of the process of listening and learning from a diverse group of yoga voices.

Honor the wisdom in your experience. As we'll discuss further in a moment, white, Western yogis often use symbols of yoga and spirituality to enhance how others see them. Your life and background have wisdom and valuable practices, and honoring yoga doesn't mean erasing your identity in favor of one that seems "more yoga." Like any philosophy or idea, yoga has evolved through contact with new communities and their ideas. We want to bring the best of our culture forward. For me, that includes a sense of stewardship over the natural world and a discerning relationship with material possession.

Avoiding yoga as performance. There's a performative aspect to yoga that we emphasize every time we say a pose "eventually" will look one way, or there are "levels" to postures. Every time we post a photo of a yoga pose to social media, we reaffirm what yoga is to the yoga community and the wider community looking in on yoga.

I'm not suggesting you should never put up photos of yourself doing *yoga-asana*, but we need to consider how, depending on our embodiment, we are participating in cultural production in a way that ignores other people's experiences.

For example, let's visit the 90s. There is a famous scene in the 1999 comedy *Office Space* that features an employee driving to work and rapping along to loud rap music. This character is defined by his aggressive feelings and simultaneous suppression of them at work.

While the employee is waiting at a stop light, a car occupied by two black men pulls up alongside him with their windows down. Our protagonist immediately stops rapping and conspicuously turns the music down, avoiding eye contact with the men in the car next to him. He gets to enjoy the outlet that rap music can provide, but without any of the collateral consequences of being African American—systemic, insidious, and overt racism in America.

White yoga teachers who adopt spiritual names and yoga costumes get to use the symbols and signifiers of spiritual authority borrowed from another culture, but also get to take them off when it's convenient. They can choose to go by their spiritual name in one space, but keep their "professional" name in others—the spiritual name is itself part of a performance of spirituality.

What makes this performative quality of spiritual authority particularly hurtful to yogis of South Asian descent is that when they offer insight from their experience, they are sometimes told their knowledge and feelings are inaccurate. That dismissal can look like a total disavowal of their experience, or the insistence that they "misunderstood" the other person's intentions. This positions the misunderstanding as the problem that needs to change, rather than the behavior.

To open ourselves up to the possibility that we are operating exclusive yoga spheres, or have misused yoga symbols, can feel shameful and awkward, but that's insufficient reason to avoid having these conversations. Collectively, we get better at having discussions when more participants are thoughtfully involved and are willing to allow for their own humanity. That is, they accept that even though they didn't intend to be hurtful, their actions may have inadvertently hurt someone else, and they are eager to explore and remediate the impact of their behavior.

It is not that you cannot talk about yoga's culture, philosophy, and history—you should! However, it's important to contextualize it with your own life and wisdom by weaving the two together. See the spiritual knowledge in your life experiences; knowledge that does not need dressing up or doctoring to be meaningful and have something to offer. My spiritual name is Kathryn—what's yours?

Spiritual Bypassing

When I failed to make a new friend in that food vendor lineup, I did not know the term for what was happening in our conversation: *spiritual bypassing*, a concept first introduced by Buddhist teacher John Welwood in the 1980s.

Spiritual bypassing is the use of spiritual jargon and concepts to avoid difficult conversations or unresolved wounds, both personally and interpersonally.

Personally, that may be feeling pressure to try to find the meaningful lesson in a traumatic experience, or express gratitude for the outcome. Spiritual bypassing on a personal level tends toward promoting a toxic positivity, and a reluctance to allow that some thoughts and feelings are challenging or painful to experience.

On the interpersonal level, it may involve disavowing someone else's feelings because they do not support the collective "lightness," or insinuating that their feelings are exclusive to them and invalid.

For example, I once attended an intensive training that was problematic on many levels. The behavior of the trainer and assistants included promoting guidelines for the trainees that didn't apply to the trainers themselves (like foregoing coffee), and criticizing the trainees to the point of cruelty.

They shouted in-the-moment feedback during our practice teaches. One training assistant would whisper unkind feedback while we were working in pairs, prompting tears from various students. When those exercises were over, the group was asked, "Wasn't that a great activity?" I was so angry and frustrated by the strangeness of this training that I raised my hand to explain that I disagreed. My statement was met with disdain. For the rest of the training, I would occasionally get called out for not actively participating.

When the assistant tried to hand me written feedback, I rejected it and said I wasn't interested in receiving feedback from someone closed off to respectful exchange. The assistant said to me, "Do you really expect they have time to talk to you? I think they're a mirror for you; reflecting what you need to take a look at."

That's spiritual bypassing—avoiding responsibility and putting the blame on the "joykill" for ruining the love and light, or rationalizing poor behavior in the name of spiritual growth. It is prevalent in the yoga community. Spiritual bypassing includes avoiding both responsibility and questioning the ethics of our actions, and builds the foundation on which systemic abuses have flourished in yoga and spiritual communities.[10]

Comfortable with the Uncomfortable

Questioning the responsible use of yoga and acknowledging spiritual bypassing is forming part of a new understanding of "getting comfortable with the uncomfortable," a phrase that many teachers retired as we grew more sensitive to the possibility of students' experiences of trauma.

Some teachers retired that phrase when we collectively grew to appreciate that people are bringing every human experience to class, and those words could be doing a number of things. First of all, that phrase could be invalidating certain people's experiences by suggesting that a more disciplined mind would simply overcome normal reactions. It assumes that all participants find safety and comfort in the feelings of their bodies, when we know that many people dissociate from bodily sensations because they do not feel safe.[11]

It also assumes that uncomfortable physical practice is beneficial practice—as we'll explore later in the book, feelings in the body are more complicated than you may know. The guidance throughout this book, and particularly in the Cueing section, are intended to help you offer encouragement and support for the challenges of practice without dictating what they should be.

As students of yoga, we know some of our experiences and stresses need healing. We all need comfort and soothing in our lives, and yoga offers us that and so much more. Our comfort zone provides this place for healing and repair and moving outside our comfort zone is our space for growth. All practice should be done with awareness, whether it is personally challenging or nourishing. If we do difficult practices without awareness, we strengthen egoic attachments to outcome.

This process of balancing nurturing and growth includes learning about other perspectives, the relationship between intention and impact, and questioning if we are excluding certain feedback precisely because it feels uncomfortable.

As these sections explored, we need to do our individual work and our work in our communities. I hope you feel committed to compassionate self-inquiry and healing, and also feel inspired when you consider that honoring a diversity of perspectives in yoga is about respectful, compassionate evolution as a community.

"Forever Student" Mindset

WHILE THIS BOOK'S INTENTION is in the service of leading yoga classes, I firmly believe that longevity to any yoga teaching requires a "practitioner first," or "forever student," mindset.

From an outside perspective, this may seem excessive in terms of strengthening the skills needed to teach a yoga class, but as yogis, we know the importance of living our yoga.

Every element of our life forms our practice—there is no yoga without your life! However, there has to be some element of formality to practice. To refine techniques for optimal practice, we have to purposefully shape our practice so that it happens at all.

What Is Your Practice?

When I first began regular yoga practice after working through my knee injury, I mostly practiced yoga at home, while simultaneously watching *Sex and the City* on DVD...and now I write books on the nuances of practicing and teaching yoga. Where our journey begins does not dictate how it will evolve!

Some yoga folks are meditators and have a long history of home practice, and others are embracing the online yoga trend, but many have never practiced at home by their own guidance. It can be intimidating to begin a home practice, especially as yoga can be an activity in which you rely on being told what to do. The journey of becoming a teacher includes refining how you practice as a student. To become a scientist of yoga, you have to wade into some uncertainty and experimentation to orient you toward the right practice.

Most of us are studying Hatha yoga, a school of yoga that is stripped of the ritualistic and magical elements of earlier forms. Hatha yoga's path to freedom (*moksha*) requires only postures (*asana*), breath control (*pranayama*), and meditation (*dhyana*). For many students in the early stages of yoga practice, these three elements form their exposure.

We've already thought about some of the ethical components of yoga practice, so let's establish your home practice for these three "on the mat" components.

You can journal throughout this section and draw up a plan for your daily/weekly practice.

Asana

To inspire a self-guided practice, you can first turn to guided online practices, which will help you get used to creating space in your home and moving your body. As you use these resources, you will gain confidence, and may choose to change or abstain from certain postures, since you have the freedom of being alone. Practicing with online classes can spark the creative juices of sequencing—if you don't like what the class is offering, then what alternatives can you come up with?

You should have some sequences in your back pocket that could be left over from your yoga teacher training, or any teaching you are currently doing. Use these to begin practicing without outside guidance. Make a point of deciding if today's practice is just for you, or if you are going to think through how you would teach the practice, allowing for cueing, duration, prop options, etc.

Begin to keep track (mentally, or with notes) of the effects of specific postures and activities, noting which poses help with anxiety, calm overexcitement, or foster inspiration. For example, your notes might look something like this:

High anxiety: Dancing Warrior (*Virabhadrasana*) series and supported Fish pose (*Matsyasana*)

Sadness: Restorative yoga with "bolster hugging" support

Excitement: Long-standing sequence with Goddess poses (*Utkata Konasana*) and standing balance play

Exhausted, but craving movement: Rolling around on the ground with moderate hip and core work

These notes will help you learn that it's not about one practice evolving into another, more superior, practice; all the tools of yoga are available to you for meeting the needs of today.

Breath Control (Pranayama)

Technically, *pranayama* is any time we choose to breathe consciously. You have many formal practices to choose from (as described later in the *"Pranayama"* section), but even if only for a couple of minutes, make conscious breathing a regular part of your practice. The best way to overcome the "imposter syndrome" that can accompany teaching unfamiliar methods is to just start working with them! *Pranayama* does not need to be fancy or elaborate, but just like any practice, aim for some consistency.

In your daily life, take notice of when you find yourself holding your breath throughout your day, and make an effort to start taking purposeful breaths before speaking and acting. You could make it a habit tied to another action, for instance, breathing consciously every time you get in the car, or before you send a text message (an affirmation on your dashboard or in your workspace that reads "BREATHE" could be helpful!).

For formal practice, make a plan using the *"Pranayama"* section. For an example, see below.

10-Minute Pranayama Practice

- 4 minutes *Dirgha Pranayama* (warm-up)
- Two rounds of 30 *Kapalabhati* repetitions (digestive fire (*agni*) stoking practice)
- 3 minutes of *Nadi Shodhana* (smoothing out the *prana*)
- 1 minute of observation/integration

Meditation

Some people who come to yoga teacher training have a consistent meditation practice they have had for decades, and others are intimidated when they discover the course will include meditation.

Meditation can be intimidating because it can seem very severe and intense, but in truth, the patience and self-compassion with which we approach meditation *is* the practice. It is simple, though it can be challenging to start, and it does get more comfortable with time. This process is the cultivation of *sattva,* the quality of lucidity, peacefulness, and illumination.

There are many approaches to meditation, but one of the most helpful mindfulness meditation techniques is *labeling* or *mental noting.* You sit quietly and steadily, observe the movement of breath in your body, and endeavor to anchor your mind to that movement. When your mind wanders, you note the content of the thought for what it is: *escapism, planning, analysis, judging, fear, story-telling, nostalgia,* etc. Once you categorize the thought, you let it go and return to your breath.

If seated meditation feels too intimidating, here are other techniques you may want to pursue:

* Walking meditation
* Guided meditation
* Mantra recitation or chanting *(japa mantra)*
* Yoga Nidra (guided yogic sleep)
* Mindfulness techniques (workbooks, coloring, etc.)

- A *pranayama* practice
- Yin or restorative yoga

There are ten *Upanishads* ("sitting down near") texts that are filled with wisdom on the nature of reality. In the Brihada-ranyaka Upanishad, the main figure, Yajnavalkya, describes the fabric of universal reality as "woven warp and woof."[12] In woven fabric, the warp threads run vertically, and the woof threads run horizontally, together they make strong fabric.

When we meditate, we want to create a clear container for practice with defined boundaries. Without defined boundaries, we will struggle to develop consistency. While there is value in occasional meditation, to be sure, consistency offers richness and deeper rewards. Consistency over time forms the warp and woof of meditation practice, making a strong fabric.

1. Create a meditation spot
It is most helpful to have a specific spot set up for your medi-tation practice, but anywhere will do. A meditation stool, cushion, or simply a pillow and a clean corner is all you need. You could sit in a spare room, bedroom, or any place where you can sit in silence (I know someone who chose to sit in her closet because it was the only place she could reliably be alone). If you have time and space, make a little sanctuary. Creating a space for dedicated ritual is a part of our spiritual practice, and tidy space reflects the goal of tidying up the clutter of our mind. Even cleaning the space in preparation for meditation is an act of devotion to ourselves.

2. Decide when you will meditate

Sometimes you need to decide when to meditate spontane-ously, but be routine if you can. Beginning with five minutes in the morning after waking and at night before sleeping is a good start, but sometimes family or work schedules require lunch-time meditation. Commit to your time and consider tracking your efforts. Inform roommates, spouses, children, dogs, etc., that you will be meditating at this time and need to be undis-turbed (and turn your phone off!).

3. Use a timer

Have you ever found that self-directed integration practices, like *Savasana* or restorative yoga, can be fraught with wonder-ing how long you should stay in the pose? When we meditate, building our container for practice includes setting a timer, if we are not practicing in community where someone else su-pervises the time for us. You can use the timer on your phone (or another alarm clock), but place it behind you to remove the temptation for peeking. If you are trying to place boundaries on phone use, choose a plain timer to reduce the temptation to return to phone use after meditation.

The Insight Meditation app timer has many free meditations for you if you prefer a guided meditation, but you can also set it to track your own meditation. It even includes punctuation bells to tell you how far you are through your sit (some people find that helps them focus, and some people prefer to just flow start to finish).

4. Always a good sit

We unnecessarily judge meditation and yoga practices as good or bad. Some days it may feel like you enter the flow more naturally, and some days your mind will put up a lot of resistance that you experience difficulty. Remember, both are good. You did the meditation, and regardless of your feelings about the practice, it was a good practice.

5. Be kind to yourself

Sitting with yourself can be quite a challenge—we get very good at what we do all the time, and if you don't take time to self-reflect often, you may be unaccustomed to this way of being. It takes time to become comfortable with it, but it happens. Be gentle with yourself in practice and in the words you use to describe it.

In many ways, the yogic journey is the journey of learning to be alone with yourself. That can be as straightforward as learning to meet your own exercise needs with *yoga-asana*, and as profound as finding inner peace.

Activity

If you are someone who likes to acknowledge their commitment with tracking, visit www.kathrynanneflynn.com and find the "Daily Effort" calendar under "Printable Downloads."

The Yoga of Your Life

One of Susanna Barkataki's suggestions to honor yoga is to "recognize your positionality," which means the social and political context of your identity. I think one of the reasons that white yoga practitioners often appropriate the aesthetics of Desi cultures is because they do not see the wisdom and spirituality in their own life and culture. Granted, our capitalist culture is one that extracts every cultural expression for its saleability, but in our individual lives and heritage, there is both wisdom and beneficial practices. To bring those into your yoga is part of the practice. For example, I live in the woods and find myself a steward of trees and wildlife. I cannot observe their changes and behavior without making a connection to my spiritual life. I frequently bring these observations to my teaching.

In your yoga journey, you will experiment with different tools to see how they help you and your students. The tools of yoga look like practice techniques of *asana*, *pranayama*, and meditation, in addition to ideas about how to live your yoga. If you study Ayurveda, your tools might become oils, herbs, and lifestyle routines. Some tools will accompany you on your entire journey, and others you will retire as your scope of understanding evolves. The tools you pick up are just pieces of content, and their intention is typically to be helpful—though no tool is universally beneficial to everyone who tries to use it. Sometimes we pick up a tool that we think is helpful—our intention is good—but then realize later that the impact the tool had on our practice was not good in the end.

Spending time with yourself to determine your core values—defining what is important to you in words that resonate with you—will help you orient your action in the world. I revisit this activity occasionally and am always interested to see how some core values remain steady, but the goals they inspire change over time.

By doing this activity and studying yogic texts and practices, you will have a clearer vision of how yoga comes alive in meaningful ways in your life.

Journaling Activity

Take a few minutes of journaling to begin your exploration of personal ethics. What is it that drives you? What is it that you are trying to realize in this lifetime that yoga is helping you to be? Kind? Calm? Rich in family? Material security?

Write down your thoughts and at least three to five core values. If you need some inspiration, visit www.kathrynanneflynn.com and find the Core Values Worksheet under "Printable Downloads."

Mantra and Affirmation

From yoga's texts, we receive a system that seeks to end personal suffering by applying techniques and embodying ethics. These methods and beliefs help us to rise above over-identifying with our ego and failing to align with our "higher selves": ourselves as part of the cosmic order.

Interpreting the texts of yoga includes studying commentary and history, as well as considering how the concepts address the specific needs of your life. Historical interpretation gives us context, richness, and direction, but there is also a modern application, which breathes new life into ancient practices. *Mantra* and affirmation practices can bring yogic concepts into your daily life.

Mantra

Mantra is a compound Sanskrit word that can be translated as a "vehicle for the mind" (*manas* = mind and *tra* = vehicle). *Mantra* can also be translated as "that which saves the mind" (*manas* = mind and *trayati* = to liberate).

Mantras are specially energized sounds, words, or phrases that are recited in a regular/repetitive manner to achieve psychological change. *Mantra* as a practice is an excellent preparation for meditation, as it harnesses the senses and focuses the mind (*manas*).

To develop a *mantra* is a very natural human thing to do. We have all kinds of beliefs and patterns built on them—we hold all kinds of *mantra* as *samskaras*. In the same way that we give our bodies regular, regimented exercise, we should give our minds regular, regimented exercise of *mantra*.

You can also think of *mantra* as the tool you apply to relieve yourself from excessive thoughts, in the same way you have your techniques for alleviating a sore muscle.

Japa (literally "muttering", but also repetition) is the practice of reciting *mantra* like a meditation. It is often practiced with a *mala* (garland), similar to the basics of a rosary, which is a string of 108 beads draped over the middle finger and held at about heart level. Using your middle finger and thumb, you pass over a bead for each repetition of your *mantra*. Infusing your practice with intention is important, which makes this meditative practice more potent.

You could choose a *mantra* that is familiar, like *OM* or *Ahim Prema* (I am love), or you can choose something more elaborate.

Affirmations

The words *mantra* and affirmation are often used interchangeably, but we should think of them differently. An affirmation is a positive statement that connects you to your core values.

Affirmation practice is powerful, as evidence by research at Carnegie Mellon University that examined students' performance in high-pressure, problem solving-based exams after taking their history of stress.

Results showed participants who were under high levels of chronic stress during the past month had impaired problem-solving performance on exams, correctly solving 50% fewer problems than students who had not experienced chronic stress.

The students who experienced chronic stress were given the opportunity to go through a self-affirmation exercise that helped them connect with their highest values, like the previous section's activity. The exercise so negated the deleterious effects of stress that the students performed as well as their less-stressed peers when tested again. Outwardly we are more likely to achieve our goals if we connect with our intentions.[13]

This has an internal affect, too. Another Carnegie Mellon study had students participate in a self-assessment exam to explore the gap between what people say their morals are and what their actions reflect. The study cited previous research demonstrating that acting *out* of alignment with what we say we value causes us distress, consequently prompting us to engage in justification techniques, such as revising or reinterpreting history, to diminish that distress.

The experiment was this: would the mere mention of morality via the Ten Commandments influence the honesty of the participants? The exam included mentions of the Ten Commandments, so participants were not being specifically cued to think of their self-described morals. At the end of the exam, the students graded their own results. The results were clear: even subtle reminders of morality inspire moral behavior. When the Ten Commandments were simply mentioned, participants were honest in their self-assessment. When the Ten Commandments were excluded from the exam, participants were more likely to be dishonest in their self-assessment.[14]

So, what we can take away from that experiment is that we can either bend our morals to fit our actions, or by reminding ourselves of our values, our actions can be informed by them. To harness the power of affirmations, you could create a series of affirming statements and post them in places where you will see them frequently, such as your bathroom mirror, the fridge door, your car's dashboard, or your cubicle wall.

If you're feeling stuck, you could source the inspiration for your affirmations from yogic texts. The *Yoga Sutras* could inspire you to think about truthfulness *(satya),* or non-harming *(ahimsa).* The *Bhagavad Gita* could encourage you to think about right action *(karma).* You could simply post these words around where you'll encounter them naturally (though you might find that "KARMA" posted around your house may seem a bit threatening), but you could also evolve the words into intentions/affirmations inspired by these concepts, specific yoga *sutras,* or passages from the *Gita,* and meaningfully work them into your daily life. Here are some examples:

On this path, no effort is ever wasted. – quoted in *Bhagavad Gita,* II.40

My perception is clear. – inspired by yoga sutra I.7

I am love. – inspired by *ahimsa,* non-violence or loving-kindness

My practice is generosity of spirit. – inspired by *aparigraha,* non-covetousness

Activity

• •

Write the affirmations clearly on paper and post them around your home/work/living spaces. Spend a week noticing their influence, and then journal your experience of trying to live your yoga, as directed by you.

PART TWO

The Bodymind

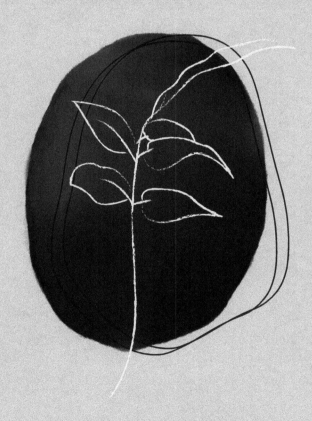

IN YOGA WE SOMETIMES use the phrase "bodymind" to discuss the inextricably interwoven system of "you." Bodymind refers not just to the material tissues and substances that comprise your physical person, but also the consciousness that illuminates it.

This interconnectedness—this union—should be remembered when we study how people move. Even if we agree that there really is no such thing as mind governing body or body governing mind, as I will try to demonstrate in this section, we must admit that teaching yoga sometimes perpetuates the idea that one dominates the other. Consider the following phrases from teaching *yoga-asana.*

Your mind controls your body.

We subtly, yet consistently, imply that we have the ability to direct our body at will through the cueing of *yoga-asana.* We use cues such as "engage your muscles," "bring your knee to your chest," etc.—as if you were somewhere in there and your foot is some separate thing that can be commanded with an on/off switch.

Of course, these kinds of cues are necessary to convey physical movement or activity through language (a totally different system of expression), but you can also see how this language reinforces the idea of the ego as an "I" center of command, dictating directions to an obedient body. When your body does not obey your commands, it can cause frustration or feelings of failure.

What is important to remember is that sometimes the control is just not there right now. Your brain sends electrical impulses to nerves that enliven tissues, creating contractions or promoting relaxation. As we discussed earlier, sometimes the appropriate motor units do not activate, and our movement practices are trying to train these connections.

Your body controls your mind.

Conversely, we imply that our body is doing things to us when we use phrases like "my back is killing me," as if your back muscles are a separate entity causing you pain.

When you move, your muscles—their range, control, flexibility, and strength—are influenced by the interplay between your body and your nervous system, in all its complexity. Your nervous system is defined not just by its material makeup and designated functions, but by its "plastic" nature—plastic in the sense that it can change, and has changed over the course of your life based on your experiences.

Your body also communicates back to your nervous system. You have sensory receptors throughout your body that convey information about physical stimuli (including external pressures and temperatures) back to your brain. (Fun fact: your skin has sensory receptors for temperature, but not for wetness, which is why you can sit on a wet chair for a while before you feel cold.)

There are also chemical messengers such as hormones and neurotransmitters that are produced by your body. These messengers travel to various destinations around your body and produce signals that our nervous system interprets, such as signals to stop, react to something, or move.

Any coffee or black tea lover will be intimately acquainted with the effects of the neurotransmitter adenosine. Like all neurotransmitters, adenosine is looking for the right receptor—receptors exist in the brain and body. When a substance finds a compatible receptor, they fit together and some resulting thing happens. If there is no receptor or no chemical messenger, the "thing" never happens.

For example, when adenosine floats along and adheres to its matching receptors in your brain, you get tired and are able to fall asleep. Adenosine is a by-product of your muscles, which is one of the reasons that exercise helps you sleep!

You probably know that caffeine is a stimulant—the reason it prevents sleepiness is because it is the same shape as adenosine. It binds to the receptors that adenosine should bind to, which blocks the adenosine from binding.

There are all kinds of similarly informational substances floating around your body, telling you to relax, causing your pupils to dilate, and directing blood to concentrate in one area of your body over another. All kinds of actions are happening behind the scenes, beyond the brain's issuing of commands.

These processes should remind us that the conscious mind does not have the whole picture; it needs feedback from your body—and that feedback may be so subtle that you need to get quiet, attentive, and take some things *off* your to-do list in order to hear the message. It really is a loop, the bodymind, and so moving our bodies and being aware of what is happening in our bodies (even if it does not consciously register) harmonizes you on so many levels that you are unaware of.

Change is Possible

Neuroplasticity

YOGA PRACTICE IS BOTH a deconditioning of the mind and a conditioning of the body. Both processes rely on one of the more exciting discoveries in the field of neuroscience in recent decades: *neuroplasticity.*

Historically, the brain was believed to be fairly rigid, and entrenched behaviors and intellect were viewed as unchangeable. However, research, particularly into the brain/movement continuum, has now demonstrated that we are in fact very capable of changing our brains. This ability to change is referred to as *neuroplasticity*, the brain's ability to change its form and its function by allowing certain pathways to fall dormant, new ones to generate, others to solidify, etc.

The theory of the unchanging brain arose out of a belief that brain development (neurogenesis) only occurred during infancy and childhood, when brain wiring occurred only during critical periods of growth. People who suffered brain trauma and abnormalities were told to learn how to cope within their limitations, particularly because they rarely fully recovered lost abilities. Scientists were unable to study the brain well, and adopted a mechanistic view of the brain, which remains somewhat present in language related to computers and wiring.

While it's true that childhood is the time of greatest brain development, we actually maintain our ability to develop new connections throughout life. This forms the basis of Hebb's Law: Neurons that fire together, wire together. Conversely, neurons that fire apart, wire apart. Neurons that fire together form a neural network, and the more a thought, feeling, or action is repeated, the more easily those neurons fire together simultaneously. Remember those "grooves of the mind"—*samskaras*—we discussed? In neuroplasticity work, science caught up with what the yogis knew.

The ability of one neuron to excite and "wire together" depends on the strength of their synaptic connection.[15] If you want to create change and strengthen synaptic connections in your brain, whether that is being a more compassionate person or honing a range of movement, you have to introduce a practice that will exercises the necessary connections and do it consistently over a long period of time.

Yogis know this, too, if you look back to the Yoga Sutras of Patanjali chapter 1, verses 12-15. Of particular note is sutra 1.15, *"This practice becomes firmly rooted when it is cultivated skillfully and continuously for a long time."*[16]

Yoga can have huge benefits on various levels, and ancient yogis identified habitual thoughts and behaviors as beneficial or harmful patterns (*samskara*). The more we engage in a certain pattern that strengthens a particular neural pathway, the more likely it is that that pattern becomes the default, and is thus more likely to happen automatically.

Motor Learning

Neuroplasticity has huge implications for the study of movement, but even though it's an exciting development of modern science, it isn't always a beneficial trait. Toronto-based psychiatrist and researcher Dr. Norman Doidge termed this "the plastic paradox": Neuroplasticity can help us change, but it's also responsible for some of our tendencies toward rigidity and sticking with more-harmful entrenched habits.[17]

That paradox includes some movement patterns, which may have evolved to keep us moving and living our lives, but can eventually cause movement restrictions or injuries. Undesirable movement patterns can be re-trained just like any other *samskara,* but we may have to be patient—the deeper the groove, the greater the effort required to change it.

To change a movement pattern, we have to put in moderate effort over time—a balance of consistency and longevity (see the section on Mapping Movement for more information).

There is a place for intensity of practice, such as a 40-day challenge, a retreat, or training, but what is more impactful is the practice we develop and can sustain over time.

For example, if you want improved hip mobility, you need to do your hip mobility exercises with some regularity over an extended period of time in order to see change.

Science backs this up. Neuroplasticity researcher Alvaro Pascual-Leone[18] discovered that neuroplasticity is a two-stage process. In the first stage, we rely on existing neural connections to perform a task and we moderately increase our skill level for a short time. Think of how many times you crammed for an exam, but forgot most of the information once the exam or course was over.

In the second stage of creating change, new neural connections are formed through "dendritic sprouting and arborization"—growth that takes more energy, but creates more permanent change. This process is consistent with what we know about "motor learning theory," which describes how we acquire new movement skills.

Here's a fascinating fact: meditation helps grow the region of your brain responsible for empathy, making it a required practice on this path toward "union." Exercise also helps the brain grow and develop in areas such as memory, self-regulation, mental flexibility, and learning.[19]

Consider how applicable the components of motor learning theory are to yoga practice:

- Change happens in stages (*change over time!*)
- Variable practice is important, so there are changes to the way the same movement skill is executed (*look at the same* asana *or activity different ways!*)
- Motor learning involves the learner in the process of goal setting (*talk to your students and prompt questions of personal inquiry, or take a workshop approach*)

- There are many different ways/approaches to practice (*verbally walking through the steps of a task, doing part of the whole, doing the whole task*)
- Providing the learner with feedback is important so that they can recognize their own intuitive assessment of what "feels right" (*offer refining feedback and then reinforce changes with praise*)

Activity

To explore change over time, choose a movement or mobility exercise. Perform it consistently over a few weeks and notice your skill development, remembering that skillfulness includes mental state changes. How did the movement experience evolve in your body and your mind?

Proprioception,
Nociception,
Interoception,
Neuroception

BEFORE WE DIVE INTO the "-ception section," I want to make a quick note on all these terms. The suffix *-ception* implies a layering—it is yet another invitation into the fascinating complexity of bodymind! These terms give us another lens through which we can view the benefits of yoga.

Proprioception

Proprioception literally means "sense of self," and it is sometimes referred to as "body sense" or "kinesthetic awareness"— it is your ability to sense the relative positions and movements of your different body parts. Because of proprioception, you know where your body is in space without watching yourself move – it allows you to practice yoga with closed eyes. A lack of proprioception is at play when you invite a student to do strong shoulder circles while holding a block with straight arms, and their elbows bend dramatically as they move the block more than their shoulders.

We can take for granted the complexity and coordination of our movement patterns. Proprioception can be negatively impacted by gait and balance disorders, neurological disorders and disease, or chemical impairments, such as alcohol or drug use. When we cannot sense where we are in space, movement can be challenging or even frightening.

A light-hearted example would be dogs wearing winter boots. You may have seen videos of dogs moving in dramatic, silly ways while wearing them, and proprioception explains why. As the incredibly knowledgeable team at my local pet supply store told me, when dogs can't feel the ground underneath them, they don't know where they are in space (their proprioception is compromised). Dogs respond with visible panic, which could continue until they learn how to feel where they are through the boots. (You'd be terrified, too, if it felt like the ground had disappeared!)

These dogs may not be in pain, but fear, pain, and proprioception are interconnected. When you are in pain, your proprioception can be compromised, making it difficult to detect sensory input or execute a movement.[20] While the relationship between proprioception and pain is currently unclear, there are consistent correlations between specific physical pathology, like shoulder pain, and poor proprioception[21].

This phenomenon could be protective, but remains a question for researchers. What we do know is that finding ways to move that do not trigger a pain response can be beneficial in enhancing proprioception and for getting ourselves out of pain.[22]

Nociception

Nociception is the transmission of sensory information about threats from the body to the brain—in essence, it's the "Danger, Will Robinson!" of our system.

We have sensory receptors on the free nerve endings (FNE) in our bodies, which are a kind of afferent nerve that convey information from the periphery of the body to the central nervous system. When these receptors detect mechanical, thermal, or chemical stimuli that are interpreted as dangerous, you have the feeling of pain.

How these receptors fire strongly depends on context, such as a person's health, age, and experience. For example, if someone has a lot of inflammation, they have a lower threshold for nociception firing (i.e., they feel pain more quickly). Advil (ibuprofen) is effective because it reduces the inflammation that irritates our nerve endings.

If someone knows that the stimuli are not threatening or even feel good about the effects of the stimuli (such as medication delivered with a needle), they will not feel as much pain. For example, I was scared of needles as a child, and my grandmother would offer me $20 if I would unclench my arms and get the required needle. I did, and research shows that monetary rewards dull pain![23]

Our students' experience and how they feel about any given activity/situation will dictate their comfort levels. We must think about how we can create invitational, accepting atmospheres and teach in ways that invite confidence. Remember, trust takes time to cultivate, and students are learning to trust you as well as to trust their bodies. For some people, the journey toward accurate interpretation of stimuli may be a long one.

Try to make your movement cues sound more like invitations to explore, offering options for experimentation rather than "levels" and "advanced versions". This encourages students to focus on what to do rather than what not to do.

Interoception

The receptors throughout the body—in our organs, muscles, skin, bones, and so on—gather information from the inside of the body and send it to the brain. The brain helps to make sense of these messages and enables us to experience states of being, such as hunger, fullness, itchiness, pain, hot or cold, nauseousness, needing the bathroom, being tickled, and feeling physical exertion or sexual arousal. This is interoception, and it also allows us to feel our emotions accurately.

At the beginning of most of my classes, I encourage students to take a full body "waking up type" stretch, similar to a cat waking up. This intuitive and unconscious stretching and yawning is called pandiculation, which is an interoceptive practice. When you engage in pandiculation, you get feedback from receptors throughout your body, which are all conveying to your brain varying status reports: *all good, need to pee, am I hungry?*

In addition to self-regulation, interoception is clearly linked to many other important skill areas that contribute to people's success and contentment, including self-awareness, flexibility of thought, problem solving, reading social cues, intuition, and the ability to empathize with others. This reminds us that our personal practice and investment in self-care helps us be in skillful relationship with others.

While stretching is only one part of a well-rounded movement practice, it has been shown to have an analgesic effect (soothes and calms pain). Gentle, mindful practices can help people reduce their inner noise and cultivate this interior quietude.

Of course, feelings of stretch (stretch response) provide a physical anchor to the present moment that can be soothing for some and aggravating for others. There are now a variety of yoga practices that can be of service here, such as Restorative Yoga or Yoga Nidra, which use different anchors to help their practitioners be with the present moment.

Anchors give people something to consciously breathe toward and connect them to the present moment—it could be the voice of the teacher, the tangible props they are holding, etc. Since conscious breathing is extremely effective at pacifying the nervous system, in many ways we are simply choosing the best practice to facilitate it.

Neuroception

In the upcoming section on breathing, we will discuss Dr. Stephen Porges's polyvagal theory of the nervous system's operations. Dr. Porges says that the body has the ability to read a situation and motivate us toward action before we are consciously aware of our reaction—this is neuroception.

An example he uses is our response to animals we consider either safe or scary—we act in response to our feelings about situations and people in ways that are too immediate for them to be born of logic.

As yoga teachers, this is another reminder that it is good to see diversity of experience and embodiment in teaching teams and leadership, because people will feel more safe or less safe with different people. There are lots of things you can do that are within your control to promote feelings of safety in your yoga classes, but sometimes the student–teacher chemistry is not the right fit.

Stretching, Feelings, and Injury

THE COMMON PERCEPTION OF yoga class content is a dynamic stretching routine and floppy meditation (*Savasana*). In many conversations, I have been privy to competing expectations about yoga—as one person talks about the stretching, another extols the virtues of the practically impossible hot yoga classes they love.

Either way, students come to practice with their own expectations about the content of the class, and an unconscious association between the content's value and their feelings. They expect the feelings will dominantly be sensations of stretching or strengthening, and that class styles exist on a spectrum of "stretchy" to "strengthening." The expectation this section explores is the most pervasive—that feelings are equal to benefit.

To participate in the yoga-culture movement that aims to move away from glorifying deep stretching, as well as refine our understanding and evolve our teaching, we will explore the relationship between structure and feeling.

Muscle and Connective Tissue

People partially come to yoga classes because they have bodies that are moved around the world by muscles. Their bodies and muscles perform adequately enough with minimal or no maintenance...until they don't.

Many people start yoga classes because they feel that their muscles are not performing optimally and they come seeking a muscular maintenance program. Of course, it is much more complicated than that.

Muscles are not homogenous structures. Muscle tissue and connective tissue are completely interwoven down to the cellular level, yes, but they are still two different types of tissue that behave differently *in response* to loads placed on them.

In the immediate sense, muscle tissue is more active and connective tissue is more passive, though both are active in their ability to adapt to stress over time. Muscle tissues contract when the nervous system sends an electric impulse to them (neural drive). When muscles work, energy is consumed (oxygen first) and force is produced. Connective tissues do not contract at all, though they do influence how we move—more on that soon.

Three Layers of Muscular Connective Tissue

This image illustrates the construction of the deep fascia: that which contains muscle tissues and is continuous from muscle to bone. You can think of the muscle/fascia complex as tubes within tubes within tubes.

Muscles have three layers of connective tissue that surround them right down to the fiber/cell:

Epimysium: the fibrous sheath that surrounds and protects the muscles.

Perimysium: the fibrous sheath that surrounds bundles of muscle cells (called a fascicle).

Endomysium: a super fine connective tissue sheath that surrounds/covers each individual muscle cell.

This structure makes your muscles incredibly strong in their response to the loads placed on them—fascia allows the force of the contracting fibers to transmit down the muscle into the tendons and bones.

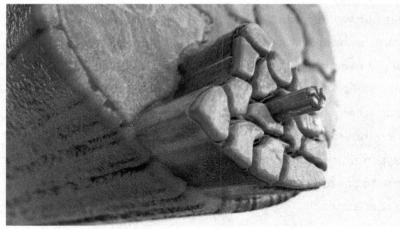

This images demonstrates the "tubes within tubes" structure of muscle cells and their connective tissue wrapping.

If you keep delving further into structure, the scale of contracting units gets even smaller. Muscle cells are comprised of structural units called sarcomeres, which are in turn comprised of proteins that change in length, causing the overall change in length in muscles. You can see that action at a macro level, like bearing your body weight in plank, also happens on a very micro level, like the changing of your muscle's proteins![24]

Motor Units and Movement

How do we go from tubes within tubes within tubes to muscle contraction? Well, next we have to look at the structural components of the muscle coupled with the nervous system.

A motor unit is composed of a single neuron and all the muscle cells it innervates. If there are fewer muscle cells associated with a motor neuron, the motor unit cannot produce as much force when the neuron is activated. It will produce weaker contractions.

All muscles are able to grade their contractions by activating small motor units first, then larger ones, as they require more force. To increase the strength of a contraction, larger and larger motor units are recruited (referred to as "spatial summation"). Once all the motor units have been recruited, in order to achieve further increase in contraction strength each neuron begins firing more rapidly (called "temporal summation").

Therefore, when a muscle contracts, it may not actually be contracting every motor unit that comprises it, but through training, we can learn to grade our contractions more efficiently, only using the smallest motor units required to achieve

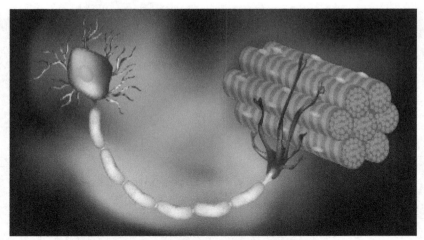

This is a motor neuron and its associated muscle cells.

the task (so, you can finally relax your face during that core sequence).

The size of the motor units in a muscle will determine the precision of graded contractions. For example, the muscles of your eyes have motor units that have as few as 10 muscle cells associated with a neuron. Your hands have motor units with as many as 100 muscle cells associated with a neuron, and your leg muscles have as many as 1,000 muscle cells in a motor unit. The eye muscles can therefore produce finer gradations of weaker contractions compared to your quadriceps, which can generate much more force, but with less precision.

Your brain does not "light up" your quadriceps when you lunge; it grades the contraction according to its prior experience. When you receive a cue that helps you discover different muscle engagements, you have likely activated your motor units more efficiently and this new experience helps build more effective motor patterns.

The number of motor units firing at any time determines contractile strength and neural feedback from the receptors, which gives you some of your body awareness. When we are training our bodies, we are actually training our nervous system, too! The bodymind is indivisible, so someone who is sedentary and does not have a movement practice may experience stiff, awkward, and unbalanced movement—the body will not perform as requested, and it feels confusing. This is part of the learning curve of any movement practice, and feelings of frustration with the body diminish as someone learns and strengthens appropriate motor patterns.

Motor patterns do not develop by activating muscles alone, but also through the enormous amount of sensory information fed to your central nervous system during the movement. A diverse movement practice looks for ways to improve those conversations throughout the body so that our musculoskeletal system functions optimally.

Stretching and the Nervous System

If movement requires the activation of motor units, what happens during stretching?

Regular movement increases our neural control—muscles contract when needed and relax when not needed. The contractions are just enough to do what is necessary and no more. The ability of the motor unit to relax increases range of movement, and regular activation increases the strength.

Passive stretching lacks the electrical impulses of muscle contractions, and it has been viewed as more mysterious and controversial in terms of what constitutes optimal practice and approach. We know that with time and effort we can adapt and remodel our tissues, since they do turn over and they do so in response to loads placed on them. Both compression loads (squeezing) and tensile loads (pulling) on connective tissues stimulate the fibroblast cells to produce more collagen fibers, which increases our fascial thickness and strength.

What we do not know is...

- How long one must hold these loads (postures) for meaningful and permanent changes to take place.
- How much is too much before we cause damage (the duration and depth of a posture differs person to person).
- How often one should be doing stretching practices for optimal gain and minimal damage.

Given the average person's yoga schedule, it is unlikely overstretching is a probable outcome over time. If someone is very frequently doing deep stretching with long holds, they may want to consider diversifying their practice.

Yogis most at risk of overstretching are those who are already very flexible and are drawn to passive stretching because they are good at it and enjoy how it feels. This may lead to chronic problems, like destabilized SI joints and knees, and they should focus more on creating stability, rather than flexibility.

Feelings of Stretching

"Passive range of movement" is the range we can access through changing position and adding loads, including the force of gravity—for example, a dangling forward fold. When we stretch a muscle, we are not actually elongating the tissue beyond the obvious length. If that seems shocking, try pulling on your finger—how long does it actually get? If musculature got longer from stretching, my hamstrings should be pooling out the backs of my legs by now! When we stretch, we are actually developing tolerance to stretch and quieting the alarm of stretch reflexes.

What are stretch reflexes and stretch tolerance? A *stretch response* is the sensation of stretching, it is what you feel when you stretch. Your *stretch tolerance* is your ability to withstand a stretch response before your central nervous system increases the alarm of your stretch response to encourage you to stop.

This design exists to protect you. For example, when you slip on ice, you might not be sure how you caught yourself, but your muscles contracted in just the right way to stabilize your balance as a kind of stretch error signal. The automatic contraction helped you right yourself and go back to a safe (non-alarming) movement pattern.

Your stretch response is a feeling of contraction that prevents you from moving into dangerous ranges of movement, but sometimes it can be conservative. Your stretch tolerance increases as you persuade your central nervous system that everything is okay, which is why you are allowed access to more passive range of movement (i.e., "further" into your stretch) when you couple it with conscious breathing. Conscious breathing calms the nervous system, which then diminishes the feelings of the stretch response.

This is also why people are able to stretch themselves into injury, because their stretch tolerance may be such that there is no "alarm bell" warning them of going so far in a stretch that they tear tissues.

Feelings Are Misleading

What is shocking about our ability to stretch ourselves into injury is that we may not even feel what was happening before the damage occurred. As we will discuss, damage does not necessarily equal pain, which means the feelings of the body can be misleading.

I think the average person assumes that, because a feeling of tightness occurs when they have not moved in some time—after a long day at the office or ride in the car—and stretching alleviates those feelings and feels good, we develop this implicit association of tightness being dysfunctional. Since the feeling of tightness diminishes with stretching, we then associate an absence of feeling with functional and safe ranges of movement.

You can have feelings of tightness and still fully be able to perform an optimal range of movement through a joint—there is nothing that necessarily needs doing. You can have no feelings of tightness, even while exploring the limits of your range of movement in your joints, and still be doing some damage to the joint capsule.

There is no need to panic—we are going to talk about injuries in the following section. This should act as a reminder of the need to cultivate inner awareness, reduce fear in our yoga spaces, and encourage people to practice mindfully and moderately.

Injury, Discomfort, and Pain

If you teach yoga, you probably have direct experience with how beneficial it can be, but you also inherently know that no movement program can exist without the potential for injury. Most yoga teachers teach the best way they know how in terms of reducing the potential for injury. Since some of us teach students of diverse mobilities, we may respond by making the practice more gentle, or creating a lot of rules around how bodies move in the service of safety.

This section tries to reposition minor injury as a somewhat inevitable part of yoga practice. While injury remains an occurrence we want to reduce, it is not always as frightening as it may seem. A yoga practice can cause some pain, but most of the time, the absence of any movement practice causes a lot more pain in the long run.

The Problem May Not Be the Problem

Before we blame yoga, let us consider team sports and desk chairs.

My partner, Alex, played a lot of sports in his youth, and has several injuries from the repeated impact of running, stopping, serving, and jumping. During nine months of paternity leave, however, Alex noticed that he suddenly had either little or no pain from his sports injuries. Paternity leave did not include much yoga and exercise (we were barely keeping it together!), but it *did* include many days with lots of walking, lifting, lowering, etc.—diversity! A diversity of movement and body positions creates optimal conditions for fewer aggravating situations in the body.

When Alex went back to work after his paternity leave, he was in pain for a few weeks, as his body grew accustomed to spending several hours a day at a desk once again. The pain from his sports injuries reappeared; not because he was playing volleyball again, but because he was sitting in one position all day long.

His shoulder injury pain became bad enough to consider surgery, but when he changed jobs and was allowed to work from home part-time, the pain dramatically subsided.

Damage May Not Equal Pain

It might be easy to say that in Alex's case, specific activities (sports) caused damage, and damage causes pain, but it is not that straightforward.

There is increasing evidence that damage to the body does not necessarily equal pain—one study showed that rotator cuff muscles (the ones that help stabilize your arm toward your body) can be torn, but still cause no pain. This study of overhead athletes (those who rely on overhead swing motions of their arms, like volleyball players) shockingly revealed that as many as 23% could have tears with no experience of pain. They were unaware they even had injuries; these injuries are thus classified as "asymptomatic"—no pain![25]

This could indicate that comfort in the body has a lot less to do with specifics than it does with a holistic ease of movement.

Your body may be accustomed to excessive sitting, running, texting, carrying children, or any number of other physical habits that shape how you move. You probably use your yoga practice as an antidote to some of the harmful effects of unconscious, repetitive embodiment—some people always want to do hip work because that's where they have tension, and other people desire more neck work because of their tension in that area. We embody in different ways, but we inhabit similar bodies—we are all 99.7% genetically identical, after all!

So, while damage to the body can definitely cause pain, damage does not necessarily equal pain. Maintaining good range of movement in the whole body, and cultivating pain-reducing practices like conscious breathing, mindfulness, guided meditation, etc., are all important elements of practice.

Connective Tissue Injuries

Knowing about connective tissue injuries is helpful to understand why we cannot stretch our way out of injuries. Injuries are more common in our connective tissue (white stuff) than our muscle tissue (red stuff).

For example, the ACL (anterior cruciate ligament) is one of the key ligaments that help to stabilize your knee joint. The ACL connects your thigh bone (femur) to your shin bone (tibia), and tears usually occur due to quick movements or impacts[26].

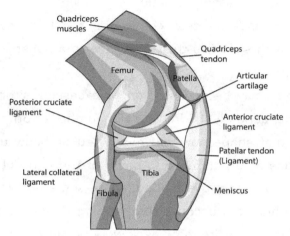

This image shows the ligaments of the knee.

Have you ever heard the joke that someone was an overnight success a lifetime in the making? That is one of the ways injuries can occur. An injury can happen in short stops or quick turns, yes, but it can also feel like it is happening suddenly when, in actuality, it took a long time for your body to create the conditions for injury.

Connective tissue can go to the end of its range of movement, after which it takes a little while to go back to its original length. Connective tissue stretched past its reasonable range is not lengthened to a permanently new length, but instead will begin to tear with micro-tears. Unlike muscle tissue, connective tissue does not repair so easily from micro-tears. People who experience ACL tears, for example, may undergo surgery to repair the tissue if they cannot sufficiently strengthen the surrounding muscles to support the damaged ligament.

A common yoga injury includes damage to the rotator cuff. Your rotator cuff is actually a group of four muscles that attach your upper arm bone (humerus) to your shoulder. The injury is called a rotator cuff tear, but it is a tear to the tendons attaching these small muscles to the humerus.

Because a lot of *yoga-asana* classes rely on postures like Downward-facing Dog as the posture around which the sequence is built, these shoulder muscles can be aggravated and possibly injured.

Downward Dog is not a bad posture, it's just that it may be practiced too frequently. Yoga classes are often built around the posture because it makes transitions between the ground and standing easier for classes with higher levels of mobility, yet we can be more creative than that.

Not All Problems Are Local

If we do not have anatomy or exercise science backgrounds, we do not always look beyond the joint or area of the body we experience pain or restriction. It's logical to address such experiences specifically, but their cause may arise from sub-optimal function elsewhere. Not all problems are local—shoulder pain can be caused by spinal muscle or hip mobility issues, and there is even evidence that pelvic floor resilience is related to the health and functionality of your feet and shoulders![27]

Individual muscles alone are not capable of moving our skeletons around, and though they obviously participate in the process, a large portion of that tensional force is transmitted via fascial sheets, where fascia transitions into one another and orchestrate holistically to create a body movement.

That is to say again, what you think might be limiting your movement may not be the obvious answer.

If you were to look at my squat position, you might say that I need to work on my hip flexibility or mobility, because I am not exhibiting an impressively deep squat.

However, you would be wrong! My hip mobility is actually quite good, but my ankle dorsiflexion is pretty limited for someone as invested as I am in movement practices.

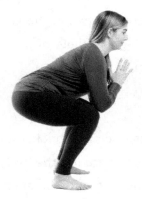 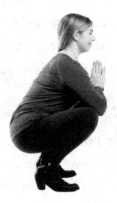

In this squat position, the feelings of limitation are in my ankles, not my hips.

In contrast, raising my heels up a few inches with boots allows my hips to flex to a deeper degree.

These photos show the difference in my squat when my heels are up, versus when they are down. In this instance, I raised my heels using shoes, but you could also achieve this effect using a rolled-up mat or towel.

Sometimes what you think is limiting you is not really a limitation, and you have to ask yourself: Does it matter? I could work on my ankle mobility, but if I am living without pain, sleeping well, and moving well, is there really a need to pursue elite movement capabilities?

The Trickiness of Injuries

Before we discuss the trickiness of injuries in plain terms in the following section, we will go through the science so you see the interplay and mystery of form, function, and the magic that is consciousness.

We discussed earlier that damage does not necessarily equal pain, but further to that, pain can be a subjective experience.

Pain begins with a signal, possibly from damaged tissue, transmitted via your sensory nerves and pathways to the cortex, where the signal is brought to consciousness. This process results in "ouch!".

Signal plus transmission equals "ouch"? It seems simple enough, but the pathways from the site of damage to the brain can alter our interpretation of the original signal. The signal can encounter certain junctions (synapses) during transmission that allow for potential modification of the original impulse—to either turn up the volume of the signal, or turn it down.

The signal goes along a pathway, with exchanges at different junctions. The original signal converts ("transduces") into an electrical impulse, which travels along the peripheral sensory nerve to the spinal cord, where it synapses with neurons that then travel to the region of the brain known as the thalamus. In the thalamus, the nerves synapse again with a third neuron that ends up in the cerebral cortex, at which point the signal becomes a conscious "ouch!".

At each junction on the way, the nerves do not only synapse with the next neuron on the described pathway, but with many other neurons, some inhibitory (turning the pain signal down), and some excitatory (turning the pain signal up). These inhibitory signals and excitatory signals determine if the original "ouch!" impulse gets amplified or dampened.

Here's the fascinating part: Our thoughts, beliefs, and perceptions influence this process. There are also pathways from the brain that descend to the spinal cord to inhibit incoming signals (descending inhibitory pathways) and these pathways are strongly influenced by thoughts, beliefs, and perceptions, and by psychosocial risk factors.

This is the reason that pain is no longer seen as a purely biological phenomenon, but a biopsychosocial phenomenon.

Biopsychosocial Model of Pain

For 10 years, my friend Geoff Outerbridge was the Clinical Director of World Spine Care, a multinational organization committed to providing underserved communities with sustainable, integrated, evidence-based spine care. Lower back pain is one of the leading global causes of disability, and World Spine Care has a yoga project component of the organization because yoga is an evidence-based approach to reducing lower back pain.

In his work, Geoff emphasizes the biopsychosocial model of pain assessment. This model does not assume the pain is a message purely born of tissue damage. Instead, pain is "viewed as a dynamic interaction among and within the biological, psychological, and social factors unique to each individual."[28]

How someone feels about their pain, the people treating their pain, their likelihood for recovery, the realities of their life and its burdens—all of these factors play a strong role in determining how people experience pain.

Negative states of mind can make pain feel more painful. As practitioner–teachers, this prompts two important things we should remember.

The first is simple: As a facilitator, you aim to create non-competitive spaces and non-prescriptive experiences (not telling people what a pose "should" feel like), and a calm environment. Reducing fear in your yoga class is important because we now know that *how someone feels about their body-mind* strongly dictates their experience. If you are listing every contraindication you have ever heard for every activity, you end up promoting the idea that much more could go wrong than right.

The second important thing to remember is that in the yoga space, there are many elements that are out of the teacher's control. These elements are not your responsibility. You cannot "save" people from their experiences. Instead, you are creating a space for them to develop skills they can use to navigate their own life. As my teacher Mona would say (quoting a gaming and lottery regulatory body): "Yoga teachers: *Know your limit and play within it.*"

Beyond the yoga classroom, how we engage with the world, in both our immediate and broader communities, is a part of our yoga. If social inequity leads to poverty, which then creates physical and mental suffering, how can you help address injustice? If we teach yoga because we believe in the healing benefits of yoga, we can stay open to the possibilities that our yoga is much more sociopolitical than we initially imagined—it is the biopsychosocial-*political* model of yoga.

How Do You Feel About Your Pain?

The bodymind can never be underestimated, just like our biopsychosocial model of pain. How you feel about a movement even dictates some of your strength, which is the basis for sports psychology.

I have seen students attempt inversions like headstands and handstands without having the prerequisite mobility and familiarity with technique—they often tumble out. If they are young and confident, feel relaxed about movement, and feel supported in themselves, they may keep trying until they develop a technique on the way up...and the way down.

These yogis are less likely to be injured, not just because they are young, with bouncy, juicy tissues, but also (in part) because of their confidence around movement and recovery from injuries.

We all have internalized stories and biases (*samskaras*) about our abilities, even if we have not consciously articulated these biases.

The same people who are willing to try a handstand without hesitation likely have other areas of their lives where they feel vulnerable and shy away from attempting certain things. As dangerous as too much zeal can be, feelings that our body has failed us, or is unreliable, heightens physical sensations of discomfort and pain. As facilitators, again, we can establish a non-competitive atmosphere and encourage people to explore their experiences without being prescriptive about what that experience should be.

Activity

Over the next few weeks, explore a biopsychosocial approach to practice. Make a point to note what is happening in your life and how you experience movement on your yoga mat. Do you notice a difference between pain or ease feelings depending on how challenging or easeful life is feeling?

Journaling Activity

Depending on your background and familiarity with anatomy and physiology, these conversations may feel "above your pay grade" as a yoga teacher. I'd like to offer encouragement—now that you know that pain can be amplified or dampened by our social experiences, you certainly have the knowledge to create supportive yoga spaces. Let's reflect on the connection between setting and experience.

Write down yoga spaces and experiences where you have felt welcome and comfortable. What were some of the specific actions that the facilitators did to make you feel welcome?

What was a time where you did not feel welcome? Was there a connection between your experience of the facilitators and the content?

Breathing

AYURVEDA EMPHASIZES THAT HOW WE DO something contributes to the outcome's qualities. It is not just what you eat, but how you eat it; not just the *yoga-asana* you do, but your energetic approach and intention. Such is breath! Many people have never considered that they should breathe differently, but hopefully they will once they land in your yoga class.

Our general inability to breathe *well* is caused by inexperience, tension accumulation in our breathing musculature, and our respiratory and circulatory systems' adaptations to the circumstances of our lives.

Breathing is the process of drawing in and expelling air, and that's a good thing, because you take an average of 20,000 breaths a day. Imagine if you had to supervise every single breath consciously—everyday activities like streaming Netflix would suddenly get a lot riskier.

Breathing is a component of the autonomic nervous system, which means that it is automatic. It is also the only automatic function that we can optionally control. We can consciously breathe and override this automated process, but for many yoga practitioners, their yoga class may be the only place this happens.

Why Do You Breathe?

Your brainstem governs breathing cues, as it is the oldest and most critical part of the brain. The brainstem's drive to cue breathing is what determines whether someone is considered brain dead or not—that is how crucial it is to live. The brainstem controls the respiratory rhythm, which is the rate and depth of your breath.

You likely think that you breathe in because your system is monitoring oxygen. In fact, it is more closely monitoring carbon dioxide (CO_2), the accumulation of which signals the phrenic nerve in the brainstem to contract the diaphragm, "inspiring" a breath (pun intended). Levels need to be monitored to ensure homeostasis, the optimal state of functioning in the body, and monitoring CO_2 levels triggers changes in breathing to regulate oxygen levels depending on what you are doing. (Oxygen levels can require a response, but the variations in CO_2 that motivate breathing changes are subtle compared to oxygen levels, which must be dramatically lower.)

Oxygen is the fuel for your muscles, so when you exercise, your respiratory rate picks up, along with your heart rate, to deliver the first fuel (O_2 being carried by your blood) to your muscles. Since you do not need to shuttle oxygen rapidly to your musculature during restorative yoga, slowing your breathing down can contribute to a rising feeling of calm.

The Benefits of Breathing Well

Breathing is the gateway and guide to the exploration of our inner experience, the doorway to conscious awareness. When we are attuned to the subtleties of our body, we are more able to discern supportive spaces (*sukha*) and practices. Breathing well also helps us:

- Alleviate habitual breath restriction that heightens physical and mental tension. Accumulated tension in the musculature responsible for breathing is going to promote shallow breathing.

- Cope with unavoidable pain and discomfort. As we know from the biopsychosocial model of pain, there are a lot of complicating factors when it comes to how we experience pain, but conscious breathing is a useful tool in pain management.

- Move through physical activity with more physical and mental equilibrium and less reactivity, potentially helping us avoid injury by improving our presence of mind and body awareness (proprioception).

- Cultivate bodymind feedback (interoception), the benefits of which are numerous (refer to the earlier section on interoception if you need to).

- Tone and support the pelvic floor, which has a myriad of benefits, including preventing/alleviating muscular dysfunction elsewhere in the body. We know the interrelationship between tissues is so complex that gripping in the pelvic floor can pull the tailbone down and forward, leading to tight hip muscles that cause back pain. Even shoulder pain can be linked to pelvic floor dysfunction!

◆ Maintain a strong and supple respiratory diaphragm. As we age, if we keep the muscles of breathing strong and pliable, we can maintain our ability to cough. The ability to cough is essential for being able to overcome lung diseases like pneumonia.

What Makes for Skillful Breathing?

When we think of breathing well, the gold standard is long, slow breaths taken through the nose.

Breathing through the nose is not just something from old yoga texts—it is actually superior to mouth breathing. The hairs of our nasal passages help filter pollutants and dust from the air, and the mucus moisturizes the air as it comes into our body. Our nose is a beautiful breathing apparatus, but unfortunately, many people do not breathe through the nose habitually because of poor posture. Postural problems can arise from excessive desk work and or inattention over the decades as we age, but regardless of how we get there, a jutted-forward head position is not conducive to nose breathing.

In response to prolonged poor posture, people are more likely to breathe through their mouth. Mouth breathing is muscularly easier, but much less beneficial. Respiration therapists emphasize the importance of a long, unobstructed airway for skillful breathing—an upright head over the chest is best.

Activity

• •

Let your shoulders slump and your head jut forward a bit, the way you might sit at a computer. Breathe through your mouth and observe the movement of breath in and out. Now, keeping the same posture, try it again, this time with your lips closed and breathing through your nose. It is difficult! This is why people switch to mouth breathing when they have prolonged poor posture.

Given the diversity of approaches to *yoga-asana* and movement practices integrated into yoga classes, there are times when the most appropriate breath is the one that helps you do the work. Breathing through the mouth during a peppy or strenuous sequence is fine, and when we return to a calm portion of practice, we can invite our students to breathe through the nose.

How We Breathe

Long-time yoga anatomy teacher Leslie Kaminoff describes the "shape changes" of breathing in the lungs and abdominal cavity as akin to an accordion stacked on top of a water balloon. The lungs (the accordion in this case) change shape *and* volume during breathing, but the abdominal cavity (the water balloon) only changes shape. Your abdomen can change volume, but you have to eat or drink something, or go to the bathroom.[29]

The muscles of breathing form a pliable and secure wrap around the lungs, like a bellows—your chest's tissues are both pliable and suitably stiff. The dominant breathing muscle is the diaphragm, which looks sort of like an opened umbrella sitting up under the lungs. It is asymmetrical in shape and has spaces to accommodate organs. It reminds me of a wonky, yet majestic, manta ray.

However, the diaphragm is not the only breathing muscle. The intercostal muscles are located in between the ribs. These muscles allow us to take a deeper breath in by lifting the rib cage up and outward during inhalation (they also work to forcefully move air out during coughing or sneezing).

On inhalation, the diaphragm moves down, pulling the rib cage wider. Our muscles move our breathing apparatus, creating a vacuum, which air then rushes to fill. Air rushes in wherever a vacuum is created—in other words, when the pressure inside a space is lower than the air pressure outside. This is why breathing grows difficult at higher altitudes, because the air pressure *decreases* as you go *up* in altitude.

In the section on *pranayama*, we talk more specifically about different techniques of breathing, but I want to make one important point here. Breathing well of course requires the ability to expand and contract the musculature of breathing. Your breathing musculature obligingly fulfills its duties, like your whole bodymind, but it adapts to the demands placed on it. Musculature requires training, through increased demands over a period of time, to attain more optimal performance. However, some activities can create beneficial change today, too.

When you are tense, your shoulders round, and your respiratory muscles are not "flexing" fully, which leads to "breathing at the top of your lungs." For example, when sitting or standing, the force of gravity directs most of the pulmonary circulation through the bases of the lungs, while ventilation is occurring in the upper lobes of the lungs (for the anatomy nerds, this is called ventilation-perfusion mismatch). The result is that more CO_2 is produced by the holding of tension, while less CO_2 is cleared.

You can train the breathing musculature to improve in strength and pliability, just like the rest of your body. It is important to move and stretch the muscles of the head and neck, shoulders, back, sides, and abdomen to promote good breathing. These are not just activities for classes with older or lower-mobility students, because remember, someone could look muscular and lean and yet still suffer from the many side effects of poor breathing.

When you are teaching mindful breathing, your cues should include relaxing any tension in the head, neck, and shoulders to promote beneficial volume on inhalation and complete emptying of the lungs on exhalation.

I should note here that, in actuality, it is impossible to completely, fully empty your lungs. However, your students really do not need to be told this because it *feels* like your lungs are empty, and that is good enough for an in-class context.

Your Voice and Your Breath

Vocal coaches will tell you that a good singing voice is a balanced singing voice—one where the vocal cords are neither too weak nor too strong, but supple *and strong* (sound familiar?). A weak singing voice may have airflow before the sound comes out, resulting in a "breathy" voice. If you tend to attack the first note of an OM chant, your vocal cords may be too strong or rigid.

Your vocal quality is intimately related to your breathing ability in that the structure of the lungs and throat influence both. The larynx is the part of the airway that divides the upper and lower respiratory tract. The larynx contains the vocal cords, two bands of smooth muscle tissue, and the opening between them is called the glottis. Sound or voice is produced when the vocal cords vibrate as air flows outward during exhalation.

We may think of the ability to allow air to flow out an open glottis as important, and it is. However, ensuring the glottis can close is also important as we age. The ability to close the vocal cords is important in generating a strong cough, which can help your lungs fight off infection.

Breathing well will help maintain the structure of your lungs and throat, but singing and chanting help as well. Yoga for seniors should include some kind of exchange—speaking or singing—as many seniors' vocal cords deteriorate because of social isolation and excessive silence. These are fun ways to exercise breathing musculature, but the most fun may be laughter yoga – HA HA!

Respiration

Breathing is the action of air moving in and moving out, but respiration is the chemistry that happens within your lungs. Let's now turn to the gaseous exchange between breath and blood.

What do you think the majority of our atmosphere is composed of? I know I had the impression that we're all breathing in oxygen, but the atmosphere is actually just over 78% nitrogen, which benignly moves in and out of you. As your heart pumps, it circulates blood that comes into contact with the air in your lungs. Across thin walls of tissue, oxygen diffuses into blood that is pumped out the left side of your heart to circulate through the body. Blood carrying carbon dioxide, after the oxygen has been absorbed, returns to the right side of the heart.

There is about 21% oxygen in the atmosphere, and it saturates our bloodstream at just the right amount, all the time. (Beyond nitrogen and oxygen, there is a small amount of argon in the atmosphere, and even less of carbon.) Oxygen is the fuel for our muscles, so when you increase your musculature exertion, your heart rate rises and more oxygen is delivered to your blood. As long as you don't have a condition that limits breathing, your body beautifully manages the oxygen meter for you.

A Radical Breath Suggestion

In yoga classes, "three-part breath" is the typical approach to teaching conscious breathing, which we discuss in the "*Pranayama*" section as "the long breath" (*dirgha pranayama*).

In three-part breathing, students inhale to expand the belly, the ribs, and the collarbones, before reversing the process on the exhalation.

I'm going to suggest something radical: consider focusing less on belly expansion when teaching your breathing. Because so many people have less than the ideal range of movement to the musculature of their chest, they overemphasize the belly movement of the breath. The same people may lift their shoulders or "pop" their chest up when they breathe (because they're trying to breathe fully), but limitations in the chest muscles cause compensation elsewhere.

As we explore in the "*Pranayama*" section, I prefer to focus on "round" breathing: breathing that expands the chest from side to side and front to back. Yes, the belly will expand, but with less focus on the belly expanding, we focus the attention on where we want to train, rather than on the path of least resistance.

Another way of thinking of this is "four square" breathing, which is my most frequent breathing cue and, when practiced subtly, is an integral part of many meditation systems.

The cues are simple and evoke the shape of a square: Breathe In—Pause—Breathe Out—Pause.

Breathing and the Pelvic Floor

When you breathe in, your diaphragm moves downward and flattens, and when you breathe out, it lifts and moves upward. Your pelvic floor—the group of muscles that sits at the base of the pelvis—follows the diaphragm. Not only does diaphragmatic breathing (the term for breath that maximizes the use of the diaphragm) stimulate the vagus nerve, which promotes relaxation, it also helps to tone and relax the pelvic floor muscles.

As I discuss in other sections of this book, for musculature to be considered functional, it should be able to contract, lengthen, and relax. An inability to relax the pelvic floor muscles can lead to the dysfunctional evacuation of the bladder and bowels. When we cannot pee and poop properly, all kinds of trouble can arise that increases our suffering.

After my pregnancy and labor, there was significant, though unfortunately typical, damage to my pelvic floor. It felt like part of me was going to fall out of my body, and it was diaphragmatic breathing that was a significant part of my recovery. Remind your classes: Breathing well helps us to poop well, and pooping well is essential to happiness.

Polyvagal Theory of the Nervous System

One of the most consistent and essential elements of a yoga practice is conscious breathing. Conscious breathing can alleviate depression and anxiety by restoring balance to the biochemistry of the brain, raising levels of feel-good hormones like oxytocin, dopamine, and prolactin, and lowering levels of cortisol, the stress hormone. This interplay of the nervous system and the endocrine system, which helps regulate biological functions by producing hormones to start and stop bodily processes, is a fascinating relationship. Understanding how the nervous system works helps us understand why yoga is effective for learning self-regulation.

Remember the earlier section on neuroception? It's a part of the polyvagal theory of the nervous system, which explains that the body has the ability to read a situation and motivate us toward action before we are consciously aware of our reaction. This reminds me of yoga's philosophy concept of "higher and lower selves"—that there are levels of awareness, and through yoga practice, they function in greater harmony.

Let's look at the levels of the nervous system—how they've typically been taught in yoga teacher training—and the polyvagal theory.

If your brain and spinal cord form your central nervous system, the nerves communicating with the central nervous system form the peripheral nervous system. Your peripheral nervous system has two branches to it: the somatic nervous system, responsible for voluntary control of musculature, and the autonomic nervous system, responsible for essential, unconscious functions (like breathing).

In your yoga teacher training, you may have learned that the autonomic nervous system is typically described as having two modes: the parasympathetic nervous system and the sympathetic nervous system.

Parasympathetic nervous system: your "rest and digest" state, in which all systems, including digestion and reproductive systems, are being allocated resources and attention and all things are good. For example, if you hear someone's stomach gurgling in your gentle yoga class, consider that a sign your class is relaxing! They are relaxed enough for their digestive system to be operating.

Sympathetic nervous system: your "fight, flight, freeze" state, in which non-essential systems do not receive resources—including your digestion and reproductive systems—because resources are being allocated to essential functions that improve your chance of survival. Another example from the digestion perspective: we often can't have a bowel movement when we're really busy or traveling. It's hard to poop when we have high stress levels.

The systems are often taught as being oppositional—one brings you up, the other brings you down.

We know that the body is an ecosystem and is capable of carrying out a multitude of functions at the same time, but there is still prioritization, of sorts. Since survival is critical and requires immediacy rather than thoughtfulness, we must have mechanisms to deduce danger and respond, without having to move through logical assessment.

There's a theory of the nervous system gaining interest in the yoga-sphere, as well as behavioral health clinical and research applications. It's called "the polyvagal theory" of the nervous system, and it's of particular interest to teachers interested in the behavioral health benefits of yoga.

Psychiatrist Dr. Stephen Porges is responsible for the polyvagal theory of the nervous system. You may remember that concept from when we introduced the term "neuroception" (the body's ability to read a situation and motivate us toward immediate action).

The autonomic nervous system governs how we experience the world because it is setting priorities. The polyvagal theory posits that there are not just two modes of the autonomic nervous system, but three modes, called "neural platforms."

The first is the social engagement system; formally it is called the ventral vagal complex. This mode allows us to eat and socialize. It is characterized by:

- A slow and steady heart rate
- Salivation, indicating preparation and readiness to digest
- Active facial muscles, meaning we're expressing emotions and empathizing with the emotions of others
- Engagement in prosocial behavior, including making eye contact and varying our voice tone
- Active middle ear muscles, making us better listeners

The ventral vagal complex is the state of being in which we can foster human connection. We are more flexible in our responses and adaptive to changes in our environment.

In our yoga practices, our aim is to foster optimal autonomic nervous system function with *asana*, *pranayama*, affirmations, *mantra*, and meditation, which make the social engagement system more accessible.

The second mode is still called fight or flight, formally called the sympathetic nervous system—survival mode or danger zone. It is characterized by:

- An increase in heart rate
- Blood being shunted from our core organs to our muscles, ready for action
- No or little facial muscle engagement ("flat facial affect")
- An increase in pain tolerance

The third mode is called the life threat system, formally called the dorsal vagal complex. It features us demonstrating/feeling fearfulness so deep that our life feels threatened. It is characterized by freezing and shutting down, or immobilization and death feigning.

The social engagement system—where everything is okay—is the most advanced. The life threat system is the oldest, and links to earlier brain structures as well: the "reptilian brain." We use reptiles as examples of ancient evolution, not just for their preservation of ancient brain structures, but also because their response to a threat is to freeze and feign death ("play dead").

According to the polyvagal theory, healthy individuals can move between the first two platforms with relative ease. When we are healthy, we can adjust to the circumstances.

In a yoga class setting, that looks like the arousal of the sympathetic nervous system during tricky and challenging activities or sequences, and then regulating back down to normal when the class is less demanding.

The life threat response explains why people in threatening situations do not respond the way crime shows train us to think they "should" react. Realistically, when faced with grave danger, people may react by freezing or immobilizing to save themselves, or trying to placate or comply with someone they find threatening (the "tend and befriend" strategy). In response to threatening situations, individuals often begin with a social strategy, then try a fight/flight/freeze strategy, and then "shutting down" is the last resort.

The important thing to remember is that what constitutes a threat varies between individuals and depending on a person's life experiences. As I say in the "*Pranayama*" section, there is no practice that is universally beneficial and healing—any practice can be provocative and threatening for someone.

Yoga practices can help individuals learn to move with greater ease back to the social engagement system baseline. That's one of the reasons it's important to have classes that invite students into their experiences without prescription, such as asking them to notice sensations in the body, to calm the breath as they notice, etc.

Since yoga classes do not typically offer social strategies or easy exits for self-regulating, we have to be sensitive to the possibility that some people will find class difficult because of a trauma response.

It is impossible to create a guaranteed trigger-free yoga class, since triggers can vary so greatly from person to person. A lot is out of your control. Here's some advice for managing what is within your control.

Choose music thoughtfully. There's a role for music in yoga classes, even trauma-sensitive classes, but choose with care. Avoid music with lyrics that are violent, inappropriate, or describe sad situations, like breakups. According to Ayurveda, our ears are particularly sensitive conduits for influencing the nervous system ("Vata derangement"), so we want to create a supportive auditory atmosphere.

Learn more about the body and impacts of trauma. Delve further into the relationship between trauma, the nervous system, and yoga/movement. A classic I would recommend starting with is Bessel van der Kolk's The Body Keeps the Score.

Allow for variations in *Savasana*. I know Savasana is valuable, and also that you may feel you're often trying to persuade students of why it is valuable, but remember, you don't know what people's experiences are. Imposing one way to integrate practice or moralizing stillness does not take into account the sensitivity of some people's nervous systems. You may want to offer a different supported yoga posture, potentially using props, for people who struggle with the prone stillness of Savasana, to give them some feelings of support or sensations of gentle stretch in the body to anchor their awareness. You could also suggest seated integration time, with hips supported by a zafu or the back supported against the wall.

Breathing, Hormones, and the Nervous System

Have you seen the 1975 comedy *Monty Python and the Holy Grail*? Let me spoil a scene for you. At the end of the film, the knights of the round table encounter a terrifying beast—the Killer Rabbit of Caerbannog. The rabbit (literally just a stuffed bunny zipping along a wire) prompts such fear and poses such a threat that the brave knights retreat, shouting "Run away, run away!" It's Monty Python silliness at its best! I'm mentioning it here to underscore that what the body finds threatening (thus prompting a stress response) is not always what the logical mind thinks we should find threatening.

Humans love trying to think our way out of stress. From the Ayurvedic perspective, people with a hefty dose of fire element (*Pitta dosha*) can be particularly guilty of this phenomenon—*I will think about how I would like to be, and then I will just be that way.*

As many yoga practices demonstrate, we can repattern the mind with purposeful efforts, like *mantra* and meditation. However, your body has very real responses to threats that linger in the body, responses that yoga's practices of breathing and movement can alleviate.

When you are in sympathetic nervous system mode you are more alert; in an aroused state that serves a survival purpose. You see more because your pupils dilate, you have more blood shunted away from core functions and into your muscles, so you are "warmed up" and you can respond faster (you will escape the bunny!). This is why performance nerves can actually be quite helpful, as they are motivating. Some of these functions happen very quickly because of the speed of the nervous system's electrical impulses, which stimulates a chain reaction called the hypothalamic-pituitary-adrenal axis. This axis's chain reaction is the interplay of your nervous and endocrine system. It produces a flood of stress hormones, which in turn sends the messages prompting some of these functions to occur.

The problem is that cortisol, adrenaline, and other stress hormones are chemical substances. They are not just electrical impulses that dissolve, so if they are not used to respond to a threat, they float around your system for a time until they are "taken back up" (reabsorbed by the axon terminal that released them). Until that point, you stay perpetually nervous and attuned, heightened, etc. We have far more stress in our lives than we may perceive. Driving and commuting on crowded public transit systems are both stressful activities, and inboxes are a source of constant stress, but we are acclimatized to stress so thoroughly, and we receive so little help, that we believe we are the ones who need to change.

While conscious breathing can calm the nervous system and move it away from the fight or flight response, the best way to address a high presence of hormones is to have your body use them and digest them. Exercise is the most efficient way to do that, because our aroused nervous system response naturally readies us to run (with great exertion) away from our perceived threats. That is why running is an effective way to deal with stress, whether it's from an oncoming tiger or an overflowing inbox!

Exercise is arousing in that it temporarily activates our sympathetic nervous system—it's applied stress to relieve stress—because its after-effects include regulating our response back down toward the socially engaged platform, especially when done mindfully. This is why it's important to include a "wind down" portion of class that leads into a quiet or silent *Savasana*, even if you are teaching hip-hop power yoga.

Exercise is also the best way to resolve chronic stress hormones floating around your bloodstream. While we can calm the nervous system quickly through conscious breathing and mindfulness activities, stress hormones, when released, linger in our blood for a longer time and require more effort to reduce.

Since many of us stay too long in states of constant stress, the levels of stress hormones in our blood remains high. Exercise helps us "digest" these hormones, which reduces our feelings of stress. If we have the right amount of stress and not excess amounts, we see things more clearly. Because yoga is a system for helping us see clearly and connect with our highest self, exercise is therefore a fundamental component of yoga.

The next section explores movement—the exercise component of yoga.

• PART THREE •

Movement

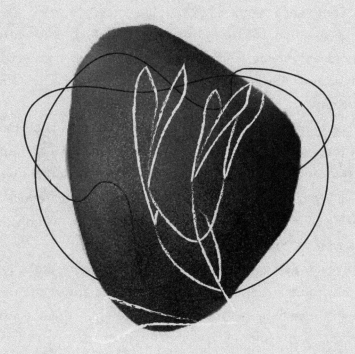

MOVEMENT CONTRIBUTES TO OUR overall wellness on multiple levels. It helps us cultivate inner calm, care for the tissues of our body, and allow for a harmonious flow of *prana*, one of our vital essences, or "vital life force."

How we choose to move in *yoga-asana* differentiates teachers and styles, and this section exists to help you understand how moving bodies work, so you see the usefulness in diversity.

Movement feels good, and generally speaking, good movement feels even better. While some yogis are keen to emphasize that yoga is more than exercise, there is nothing wrong with enjoying exercise. It is an excellent way to reduce the suffering caused by excess stress and pain. Even Swamis often had a walking practice.

However, as yoga teachers love to say, there are a lot of different tools in this toolkit. This section clarifies the use of some of those tools, so you know how to apply them skillfully.

Embrace the Mystery of the Body

IN AYURVEDA, WE TALK about the interrelationship of the qualities of the material realm (*prakriti*), that is to say, we consider how nature manifests so that through observation of it, we can live more healthfully and vitally since we are a part of nature.

In this book's section "The Qualities of *Yoga-Asana*," we explore the qualities (*gunas*) of nature. Those qualities appear to be in opposition—hot/cold, heavy/light, etc.—but it is better to think of them as existing on a continuum. Hot moves toward cold, heavy becomes light, and so on. One of these quality pairs is gross/subtle, which means some things manifest more tangibly (gross), and some things manifest in ways that are less obvious and more difficult to discern (subtle).

I think some people find comfort in anatomy because as a gross (manifested, visible) being, anatomy feels knowable and factual. When there is so much to know relative to yoga, anatomy can feel like a safe place for our egos to explore because we come out with a sense of real, concrete knowledge.

The truth is that there is a lot we know about the body, and there is a lot that remains a mystery. Some ideas in this section are more conceptual, serving as an invitation to loosen our grip on our certainty of the body. In all yogic practices, loosening our grip on certainty promotes curiosity and a little objective distance, which helps promote a compassionate lens through which we can view yoga.

Biotensegrity and Fascia

ONE OF THE MORE inspiring anatomy concepts to emerge during my yoga tenure is that of *biotensegrity*. For yoga teachers, biotensegrity underscores many of the motivations of this book: diversifying movement practice, approaching practice with curiosity over rigidity, and involving students in the discovery process.

Yoga cues can sometimes quash student discovery by prescribing feelings and outcomes that students "should" be experiencing. Cues can also promote the impression that safe movement is bound by distinct rules, the same as machinery and physics—lines, angles, stacking, etc. Biotensegrity encourages us to move away from the language of machines and buildings, and this next story illustrates the evolution of one of my cues.

Sometimes during the restorative portion of classes, I would help set up students in *Viparita Karani*—typically taught as "legs up the wall." The Sanskrit translates as "inverted," or "opposite" of "action," or "doing," so this posture and its opposite-of-doing cultivates stillness.

Once settled in, I would tell students about the Eiffel Tower. Unlike a house, the Eiffel Tower has no foundation set into the ground, the structure simply rests on top. Its materials and structure are all designed to minute degrees, allowing it to withstand pressure from the wind and corrosion from the elements—a remarkable feat of engineering.

My intention was to promote an atmosphere of ease and support, but I came to realize that I was creating a lingering comparison of bodies to inorganic materials. Bodies are not made from rigid elements, with straight lines, sharp angles, and screws connecting our joints, but that is how we often talk about them. With the concept of biotensegrity, we can begin to unravel the implications of that misunderstanding.

Tensegrity

Before we add the prefix *bio-*, let's look at the word *tensegrity*. Tensegrity begins with "tension-compression structures," sculptures by the artist Kenneth Snelson. They're made from a series of rods and cords specially assembled to build a 3D, freestanding architecture, pictured here (you might recognize these as large-scale versions of popular baby toys!).

The rods are the hard elements of the structure, while the cords run through the rods and are tensioned at the right angles. The structure then holds itself up in gravity without the need for outside support.

While this may sound just like the Eiffel Tower in some ways, the differences are that (a) Snelson's structure relies on

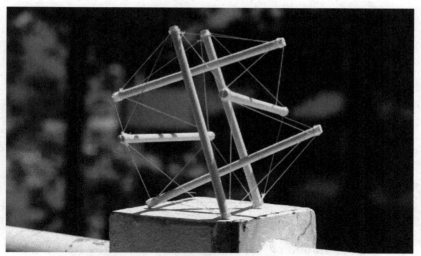

This image shows how the tensegrity structure functions.

the hard elements floating in the softer matrix of the strings for its stability, and (b) it is self-contained (no open ends). Where the Eiffel Tower is rigid in its wind resistance, Snelson's structure can bend and move without damage to the structure. A strong wind could deform it quite dramatically, and it would return to its original shape.

The tension-compression structures got a new name to describe the specific needs of *tension* and *integrity*; strings need a particular tension (*tensile integrity*) combined with the solid elements of the rods. Without that tensile integrity, a lax string affects the whole structure. This idea of specific tension and integrity gave birth to the word *tensegrity*.

There's an intuitive element to these structures. If I were to give you straws and some elasticized string, you would be able to figure out the right amount of tension in the strings while building a structure. You would learn how much tension gave it sufficient structure to stand up, but not so much tightness in one corner that the shape was uneven. You also might notice that having the right amount of space between elements improves the structure's integrity.

In the "Breathing" section, you might remember I mentioned that dysfunction in the pelvic floor can cause unexpected problems elsewhere. Think of tensegrity structures as mirroring the human body—tightness/laxity in one place over another, or an insufficiently stiff rod element, will negatively influence the integrity of the structure.

In the "Sequencing" section (in Part Five of the book), I emphasize the need for diverse yoga programming. When you're developing your sequences and style, consider some of the unconscious beliefs you might have about certain areas of the body. I've noticed over the years that yoga classes assume some parts of the body only need stretching and others only need strengthening. For example, some people with neck issues focus on stretching that area to alleviate the discomfort, but they fail to realize that the problem is actually due to inflexible abdominal muscles that need to be stretched instead. However, lots of yoga classes only include sequences to help flatten/harden abdominal muscles, not stretch them.

Like a tensegrity structure, your whole soft tissue matrix needs optimal tension to produce ideal range of movement through your joints. You need yoga that strengthens and promotes suppleness, as well as spaciousness—the components of a sound structure.

Biotensegrity

Biotensegrity uses the concept of tensegrity to better understand and express how biological tissues function in their composition.

The orthopedic surgeon who coined the term, Dr. Stephen Levin, was motivated to evolve the ideas in anatomy about movement and the architecture of the human body.

We often talk about the body's architecture as if our feet, which support the rest of the body, from the legs to the head, have the body's weight "leaning" on them.

A museum visit inspired Dr. Levin to think of things differently. As he looked at some dinosaur skeletons, he noticed that specimens like the brachiosaurus had long tails that floated behind them, rather than dragging on the ground like you might expect. If it's true that the entirety of a human's body weight is resting on the feet, then a dinosaur's tail should drag, shouldn't it?[30]

For a present-day example, you could think of a cheetah's tail, which floats behind the animal and helps it balance, rather than an extra-long horse's tail that hangs to the ground with gravity.

Dr. Levin saw a Kenneth Snelson sculpture ("The Needle") and extrapolated it to explain why bodies behave the way they do.

When you look at the Eiffel Tower, or any similar skyscraper structure, you might notice that the base is more significant than the rest of the structure—it is often more robust and able to hold up the rest of the building. When you look at nature (of which we are all a part) you see that nature defies this architectural "requirement" all the time. Trees, people, flamingos, all show us that the structure of the base is not necessarily broader or more robust than what it supports.

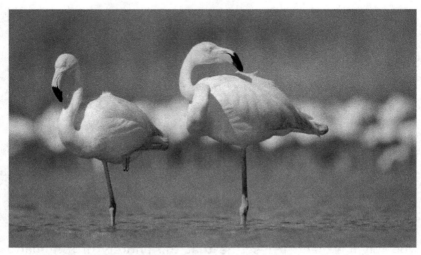

This image of flamingos illustrates how the base of a structure does not necessarily need to be broader than what it is supporting.

In many fields, including yoga, we talk about bodies and alignment as if bodies were like stacking cups—put one part over top of the other, and they support each other in response to gravity. That cannot be true, because even anatomy skeletons designed precisely to represent our skeletal shape need a rod through their back to hold them upright.

We stay up in space because we are built by roundness, beginning at our tiniest units: cells.[31] Biological tissues' cells are spherical and thus omnidirectional—there is pressure being exerted in multiple directions, not just the load of the body and gravity pressing exclusively downward onto the base. When I think of the human body's architecture, I think of a bag of oranges—roundness contained within a stretchy, yet suitably stiff material. The bag holds the oranges together, but also allows for shifting components and changes in shape that are not the least bit robotic or mechanical.

When we compare the body to machinery and architecture, we diminish the wonder of its abilities. According to Dr. Levin, if the structural principles applied to engineering governed the human body, you could break your spine by going fishing. Running would smash small bones in your feet, and picking up your child could break your spine.

What yoga teachers need to appreciate is that we are not made of inorganic matter. Tissues are adaptive; they are not just strong or just stretchy—they respond to the loads placed on them and to the surrounding circumstances. While we often have to employ metaphors to describe functions and activities, Dr. Levin emphasizes that biological tissues are not like any other tissue—they are alive. If you need a metaphor for biological tissues, silly putty makes the best one: it can bounce, stretch, deform, and reform.

The concept of biotensegrity helps explain the fullness, the unity, of movement. When you lift your arms, it may seem like an isolated action, but forces move around your whole body in order for you to make that movement, and signals are communicated to the entire structure. At the cellular level, we get stability when the opposing forces of tension and compression are even.

The takeaway is that tensegrity structures get their stability from the spaces between the elements—*by spreading out and balancing the stresses throughout the whole structure.*

Our practices of yoga are part of the equation for spreading out and balancing stresses around the body, seeking to balance strength with suppleness and provide all your structures the right amount of space.

Connective Tissue

If we think of the body as a tensegrity structure, your bones form the compression elements and fascia are the tension elements. In practical application, this means that loads get distributed around the whole structure of the body by the fascia.

As we looked at in the section on muscle cells, connective tissue wraps around all the other tissues within you, and it exists right underneath your skin (superficial fascia), as well as around all your muscles and bones, right down to the muscle fiber (deep fascia). Since we are interconnected, manipulating the skin manipulates the superficial fascia, which influences the deeper fascia. Loosely hold on to your forearm for a moment and turn your hand back and forth—you are manipulating skin, which manipulates superficial fascia, which manipulates deeper fascia. Canadian physiotherapist Diana Jacobs calls the skin "the handle" to the body for that reason, since manual therapists are never really touching anything but skin.

Generally speaking, connective tissue has three components to it. Learning the component parts of biological tissues helps us appreciate that biological tissues can do multiple things—they can be strong *or* stretchy. They are each designed for a specific need, such as support, protection, force transmission, or elasticity. For example, your ligamentum flavum (a band of tissue that connects a vertebra to adjacent vertebrae) is more elastic so as to allow the spine to flex, and tendons are designed to minimize stretch and transmit force.

The three components that make up connective tissue are:

Ground Substance: the supportive, gelatinous substance that surrounds the cells and fibers of connective tissue. Ground substance provides the right *space*.

Cells: called fibroblasts, these cells secrete the precursors required for the formation of connective tissue and various fibers.

Fibers: strands that are made up of proteins (large molecular building blocks directed by DNA), predominantly collagen and elastin, which make up 25% of your body's protein count.

Collagen gives tissues, including bone, their *stiffness*. The word is Greek for "glue producer." Elastin provides flexibility and some *elasticity* (stretch) to tissues, giving them their ability to deform and reform.

For fascia to perform optimally, these tissues rely on their ability to "slide and glide"; in other words, for the tissues to have sufficient ground substance to keep them moving without stickiness.

From the Ayurvedic perspective, aging is drying out, because the elements that govern our wisdom years (60+) are dry. Regarding tissues, as you age, your body produces less collagen (the stiff material), but the substance that allows your fascial layers to slide smoothly on each other begins to dry up too. The dryness makes the tissues a bit more grippy, which means more restricted movement.

Your tissues are like sponges that hydrate through movement; motion is lotion for the bodymind. When you squeeze, compress, and manipulate tissues, you press the water out of tissue cells, only for them to draw water back in, almost like it fluffs them back up. This is one of the reasons a good massage, or a *yoga-asana* class with a diversity of movement and activities, makes you feel good—you feel fluffier. "Soft tissue manipulation" (self-massage or massage) is also an excellent way to ensure that your fascia "slides and glides" as well as it should.

I should note that whether movement/self-massage hydrates fascia is contested.[32] However, the benefits of promoting slide and glide are not limited to muscular and connective tissue. Your nervous system's extensive network of nerves also benefits from massage and movement. When the tissues of your nerves are moved, manipulated, and stretched, they function more efficiently!

Keeping tissues sliding and functioning well relies on a diversity of movements and tempos, as well as proper nutrition to provide optimal building materials, and sound sleep for proper tissue growth and repair.

Building Connective Tissue

Earlier in the book we learned that muscle cells increase their contractile strength by stimulation via the nervous system. Neural drive (i.e., the intentional or automotive contraction of muscles) draws tension into the cells (contracts) and stimulates the cells to start adding more contractile elements (hypertrophy).[33] This is how muscles get stronger! You progressively add load, and through hypertrophy, muscles are able to generate the force to cope with the load.

Connective tissue cells respond to load added to the body by adding more fibers along the lines of force. For example, you change your position from your typical upright posture when doing a side bend, and the load to hold that new position is transmitted across your tissues. Your connective tissues' cells respond to loads shifting onto them, and with regular and consistently applied loads, the collagen organizes in a particular way with a specific density.

In the absence of optimal loading, underused connective tissue can grow weaker and less "purposeful" in its arrangement, thereby becoming more prone to injury. Think of the way produce is arranged to minimize damage—without purposeful arrangement, those apples are more susceptible to bruising. Think of our movement practices as being the produce stacker of our connective tissue—helping direct the fiber production (deposition) into a more purposeful, stronger arrangement.

Diversity of movement practice helps create load from a variety of angles and improves the robustness and suitability of our internal net.

Good movement practices help collagen fibers grow into their ideal arrangement for the type of loads that the area receives. Before we talk about flexibility, I want to clarify that stiff tissues are also vital. Stiff/strong connective tissues with sufficient springiness can absorb and effectively transmit loads, and we established earlier that transmission of load around the structure is important.

Whether we are doing strong or passive postures, the joint positions we assume and the approach we take should be in service of directing loads in purposeful ways to strengthen our muscles and connective tissue for their optimal adaptation. Moderation also plays a role, in that biological tissues develop with the right load but sustain damage with a too-heavy one.

Muscles get stronger in their ability to generate force (or bear a load) and connective tissue gets stronger in its ability to absorb and transmit load, especially turning potential energy into kinetic energy.

You can see how diversity of activity in a yoga class promotes optimal development of biological tissues. Now that we have widened our perspective on the language of bodies and tissues, we can move to discussing these activities in more detail.

Mobility vs. Flexibility

YOGA CLASS CONTENT IS always evolving. Lately, there has been a movement away from classes that are strictly traditional *yoga-asana*, and teachers are including exercises and props in the service of optimization and efficiency.

This "Movement movement" uses different terms to describe the work that they do—especially since many of these folks are trying to earn a living codifying their "specific" approach to movement—but a common term is *mobility*. Mobility is sometimes used to describe where flexibility intersects with intentional control.

Flexibility allows you to more easily move into a shape—or be moved into it—but does not offer you the ability to hold it with control, nor does it allow the ability of moving some part of your body into that position by its own power.

The familiar yoga posture known as Pigeon illustrates the difference between flexibility and mobility.

Take a moment to get into a forward folding, one-legged Pigeon pose *(Eka Pada Kapotasana)*, and observe how close your front knee and foot are to your torso. Once you have mentally marked their positioning, come into a standing position.

Without using your hands, lift the same leg toward your torso and try to replicate the proximity between your leg and torso that you noted in the folded position. Are your knee and foot in the same position they were in on the ground? Probably not even close. The standing variation reveals your hip *mobility*, the position on the ground reveals your hip *flexibility.*

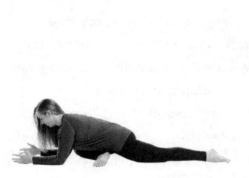
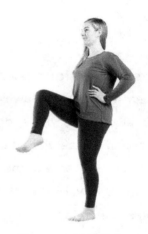

When you forward fold in *Eka Pada Kapotasana* (One-legged Pigeon pose), you are in a passive stretch that may help relieve pain, improve the efficiency of range of movement, feel relaxing, and ground the mind. This posture demonstrates your flexibility.

You cannot replicate Pigeon pose while standing, because this requires your useable ("active") range of movement, which forward folding Pigeon does not increase. This posture demonstrates your mobility.

To develop greater joint mobility, the joint muscles must train to execute the optimal range of movement. Movement around a joint relies on two set(s) of muscles, one to generate force and initiate movement, and the other to relax and lengthen across the joint.

For example, think about the action of elevating and widening your arms. Your shoulder and upper back muscles are the muscles that contract to generate the desired movement. Your pectoral muscles must, at the same time, be flexible enough to lengthen and allow the movement to happen. Without doing this specific movement at least somewhat frequently, your ability to do so may decrease (this is the reason Downward-facing Dog can be so challenging and beneficial).

By the end of this section, and before we move into sequencing yoga classes, we will underscore the importance of diversity in approach in order to promote a well-rounded practice.

Journaling Activity

Write down a long list of your specific favorite yoga activities and identify them as passive stretches (like Pigeon pose), active stretches (like Bridge pose [*Setu Bandha Sarvangasana*]), strengthening exercises, and mobility exercises.

If this were going to be your daily practice, does it require some diversification? The following section will help you modify your approach so you can develop a well-rounded practice.

Flexibility

Flexibility is the ability for a muscle to lengthen, but what constitutes optimal flexibility?

Multiple variables such as intensity, duration, repetition, etc., make stretching challenging to study, and research can become outdated quite quickly. What we do know is that genetics dictates some of our flexibility. That means that the interplay between your nervous system and tissues allows for more range of movement, and that there are some people with skeletal structures more predisposed to achieving movement without bone-on-bone compression stopping movement.

Lifestyle and movement patterns play more obvious roles in allowing for (or inhibiting!) flexibility. As the body and mind get very good at what they do consistently, movement patterns are dictated by what we do and do not do—for example, sitting, running, cycling, lifting weights, etc.

Some movement patterns can have predictable effects on flexibility. Office workers who spend most of their day sitting will likely have poor flexibility in their hamstrings and hip flexors, because both the knee and hip joints are in flexion for extended periods. Runners can get overdeveloped quadriceps groups and underdeveloped (and thus tight) hamstrings. Both scenarios can have significant impact on the range of movement around the knee and hip joints.

Some effects are more difficult to predict, like a little movement you unconsciously do all the time, but that strains your joints disharmoniously. This could be as mundane as staring out the window in one direction whenever you take break from work, or always carrying a bag or purse on the same shoulder. (However, staring out the window at work is not going to negatively affect range of movement in your head/neck/shoulders if you have a diverse movement practice.)

As we discussed earlier in the book, feelings of tightness do not necessarily indicate that musculature is suboptimal, or dysfunctional. We cannot rely on feelings of tightness as a measure of suitable flexibility.

The right amount of flexibility is that which allows you to live pain-free and move through your life with ease. Since flexibility is partially due to genetics and influenced by lifestyle, how you encourage your flexibility-promoting yoga in class will be contextual.

As yoga teachers, that means encouraging super-flexible students to balance their practice with strengthening and stabilizing activities. For yogis with the gift of stiffness, we can share that living a pain-free, happy life in our bodies does not require embodying yoga postures in certain ways. I occasionally share with classes that I live with less pain now that I do not pursue "nose to toes" forward folds.

As we will discuss further in the "Cueing" section, how we talk about embodiment, goals, levels, alignment, etc., all contribute to how our students view their own flexibility. And, as we will delve into in the "Demonstrating" section, any demonstrations should be in the service of promoting understanding, not glorifying superior flexibility. All the tools of our teaching can serve to promote the gifts of moderation.

Before You Give Up Stretching

Though passive stretching has *limits* on what it can do for us structurally, it is not without structural, functional, and psycho-spiritual benefit. Everyone, even highly flexible people, can benefit from the psychological and spiritual advantages of gentle and still forms of yoga practice. For those who already have a high level of flexibility, we can increase the restorative, supportive elements of their still practices and explore gentle, fluid movements in joint-specific activities.

Within a quiet practice, I highly recommend a blend of gentle or mellow movements throughout the practice. My belief is that the average member of the general population benefits psychologically and spiritually from a quiet practice, but the physical efficiency of a *strictly* yin yoga practice is improved when it includes some gentle movement, as well. Mobilizing tissues keeps them hydrated and springy—remember the aim of promoting "slide and glide" through fascia?

One of the most intriguing discoveries about fascia is that it is a sensory organ that plays a role in our proprioception (body awareness in space)[34] and interoception (how the body and mind connect to provide feedback on the state of "how we are").[35]

Practices that emphasize physical awareness and internal listening can help refine the sensory nature of our tissues. Preliminary studies have shown an inverse relationship between pain and proprioception, making this a worthwhile pursuit—the higher the body awareness, the lower the experience of pain in the body.

Strength, Stability, and Balance

Strength or Stability

IS THERE A DIFFERENCE between the phrases "stabilize your shoulders" and "strengthen your shoulders"? They are often used interchangeably, and even if we do not need to explain in-depth to our students, we can explore the difference here. *HOW WE USE LANGUAGE* to convey meaning is contextual— a term that conveys the right meaning in one situation could be less specific or inaccurate in another. Specifically speaking though, strength and stability mean two different things.

Strength is your muscles' ability to produce the necessary force to bear a load, whether that is holding a Plank posture, or lifting a heavy bag toward your shoulder. Right now, you can probably curl your fist and bring your hand toward your shoulder, because your muscles have the strength to do that against the load of your own body weight and gravity.

However, if I were to hand you a heavy grocery bag and ask you to do the same movement (bring your hand toward your shoulder), the load would then be greatly increased. In response to the heavier load, your muscles must produce more force to achieve the movement. If the bag were too heavy for you to lift your hand, the load is higher than the force your muscles can produce to overcome it and lift the bag.

If we took a few items out, we could add and subtract weight from the bag and continue to adjust the load until it was just challenging *enough*. To strengthen, we need the right amount of load for you to develop your force-generating ability beyond what you already possess.

Increasing load can come from other sources, too. We could also use resistance bands or yoga props to improve targeted engagement of muscles.

Props can be really helpful in teaching bodies how to engage well. The load of two dumbbells pressed overhead necessitates more obvious resistance than just reaching your hands up and "engaging your muscles." In a yoga setting, reaching a block overhead and squeezing the block will also increase the force generated by your muscles.

Reaching your hands out in front of you is the same position as Plank pose *(Phalakasana)* in yoga, but by changing our position to standing, we shift the load from one part of the body to another, and the forces of gravity act on us differently. When you hear a term like "bodyweight exercises," it refers to employing body positioning and the resistance of gravity to increase the load on our muscles. This is the basic premise of classical *yoga-asana* as exercise.

Stability is the ability to prevent unwanted movement (say it with me: *Stability is the ability to prevent movement!*). Sometimes stability is described as the ability to return to position, but this is still just the ability to prevent unwanted movement further away from the desired position than you can overcome.

What movement could we possibly be trying to prevent? The answer is *lots*—it is the basic premise of alignment.

Think of Chair pose (*Utkatasana*) cues about being able to see your toes, or the feeling of drawing your thigh bones back into their sockets when doing the posture with feet apart. These cues are meant to help students prevent their knees from knocking toward each other. The ability to prevent the knees knocking toward each other indicates stability in the muscles of the hips and knees.

You can see how strength and stability are related, but not quite the same. In Plank pose *(Phalakasana)*, you may have heard the alignment cue encouraging you to be "straight from head to heels." This cue makes limited sense from a practitioner's perspective, because their experience is so different from a facilitator's perspective.

From the practitioner's perspective, they may *feel* straight. If someone's body is sloping toward the ground and their shoulders are sagging, they are not exercising the shoulder and core *stability* to prevent that slope and sag, but they do not inherently know how to be *straighter.*

You can help students improve joint stability by providing them with feedback that teaches targeted muscle engagement in a specific context—they very well may have the strength to achieve ideal positioning, but not the awareness. In the sagging-shoulder Plank pose situation, rather than giving the student a global cue they cannot interpret, ask them to lift their shoulders off their arms a bit toward the ceiling. They can feel their shoulders and they know where the ceiling is, so you have a higher likelihood of your cues being interpreted successfully into embodiment. (For more examples on precise cueing, refer to the "Cueing" section.)

Balance

In the *yoga-asana* world, balance typically refers to a set of postures that require existing balancing skill, such as standing on one foot, one's hands, etc. Standing balances require detailed use of foot/ankle musculature and strong core muscles, but balance is technically the ability to maintain a center of gravity within the base of support, and standing yoga postures have a tiny base of support on just one foot!

However, balance is broader than that—a standing lunge is a balance posture for lots of people. Optimal balance is not just about being able to stay upright; it is about *stability* and *mobility*—the ability to not move from that position, but also to move in any direction with minimal preparation.

We can play and work on our balance skills in organic ways by working on ways of coming up and coming down, side to side, etc., in different positions.

We want to be able to move in any direction at any time, because variability and reversibility are signs of good movement. What feels like a balance posture for one person may not be for another, so our prescription for improving balance could begin at holding on to the back of a chair or the wall and lightly raising one heel while trying to center weight in the other foot.

Prerequisite Mobility

Being able to move in any direction at any time is optimal, but just not realistic for a lot of the students attending our classes.

A student in my advanced training was a flight attendant, and we were discussing the challenges she experienced with being forced to wear heels as part of her uniform. Between her predisposition toward an inflammatory condition and the exacerbating stress of a high-heeled shoe's pitch, she was unable to put pressure on her toe joints. (Full disclosure: the student and I are around the same age, so if you are imagining a senior citizen, you may want to think about some implicit associations between limited mobility and age.)

When teachers invite students to do a High Lunge pose (*Anjaneyasana*) "with their heel raised behind their toes" rather than the "back heel down" of Warrior I lunge (*Virabhdrasana I*), there is some implication that the back heel being up is the more advanced position.

It *is* likely trickier for many people (High Lunge is a balance posture, and it problematizes stability), and Warrior I can be a balance posture too, and there are many reasons someone may need a different or modified version.

What determines someone's ability to do a yoga posture with a certain alignment and qualities of good movement constitutes what I call *prerequisite mobility*: what needs to change shape, relax, stabilize, or meet a load in strength to achieve a movement.

Yoga teachers are often distracted by what a pose *might* do for someone—the most dramatic effects of the pose, if you will. We need to consider the variety of experiences people have instead, and begin to identify some of the most basic elements of a movement.

In the High Lunge example, the issue is not just the ability to balance in a lunge position, it is also the ability to bear body weight on the relatively small joints of the feet in a steep toe extension. That is a lot of weight on joints that might not have moved that way in a long time.

When students have asked for help achieving tricky yoga postures, we take the time to consider what they might need to work on specifically to fulfill the *prerequisite mobility.*

Compensation

BEFORE YOU START TO get an understanding of what may be happening, you can see compensation when observing *yoga-asana* classes. This may have come up in your yoga teacher training, with common examples like a dramatic sway to the lower back, hiking shoulders up into the ears, etc.

This is a normal, if undesirable, phenomenon. In an effort to conserve mental and physical energy, bodies often take the path of least resistance. Without proper engagement and diverse movement activities to maintain optimal joint function, bodies succumb to gravity and the loads placed on them. Over time, people may start to rely more on the support of the fibrous connective tissues (ligaments, tendons, fascia) and certain stronger muscles to carry out the function intended for other surrounding weaker musculature. For example, lower back muscles may work harder to replace an absence of strength/engagement in other core muscles (e.g., abdominals, glutes) or the hamstrings, resulting in the feeling of tightness in the lower back. This phenomenon is typically referred to as "compensation."

Nothing is inherently bad in embodiment, including compensation. Dr. Loren Fishman, a yogi-doctor of rehabilitative medicine, tried practicing a headstand when he had a rotator cuff injury that was going to need surgery. A headstand requires shoulder flexion (arms in an overhead position), but the bodyweight demands of the position were actually met by other muscles in his shoulders in a way that both caused him no pain and maintained joint strength. He was able to avoid surgery by practicing headstand and progressively increasing the load. The muscles compensating for the lack of rotator cuff muscle strength helped stabilize the joint, and his rotator cuff muscles were able to safely get strong enough again and repair the torn tissue through micro-levels of loading. (He's since successfully helped patients avoid surgery with this technique, with a success rate of over 90% of several hundred patients, using a headstand or adapted variation.)

Of course, compensation can be harmful too. Context is critical to any application of principles, and chronic compensation or overuse can lead to imbalances and injuries, like muscle strains or repetitive motion injuries. Instability in one area also affects the whole body through the ripple effect of joint functionality.

Kinetic chain refers to the interconnectedness of all joints and muscle groups in the body. During movement, joints and muscle segments affect other areas of the body, so much so that we cannot say purely that a movement, stretch, or exercise is exclusively beneficial for or performed by a specific muscle.

Over the years, I have had the benefit and pleasure of teaching in different communities and spaces with students of varying skills and struggling with a variety of challenges. Watching thousands of people moving has intimately acquainted me with the likelihoods and limits of people's movement abilities. Observation can offer you an excellent education.

Compensatory Movement Patterns

Compensatory movement patterns sometimes arise out of injuries and sometimes occur because of an inability to perform a typical movement pattern, thus causing an injury. Either way, they appear, and they can cause unexpected issues further down the road.

A compensatory pattern is the process of movement, holding, contraction, etc., that accommodates the avoidance of another joint or area to contract, and then that accommodation becomes habitual. For example, I came to yoga after developing shin splints from running that were worse in my left leg than my right. Then I got patellar tracking syndrome in my right leg because I was favoring my right side to lessen the stress and load on my left side. The muscles in my quadriceps group became overdeveloped and this compensatory pattern caused strength-based tightness that created an injury to my right knee.

Reducing Compensation Gradually

Obviously your history and your history of movement play a role in injury, but in the moment, speed, force, and positioning all play a role as well. As yoga teachers, we can cue for proper positioning instead of rules-oriented alignment, we can be mindful about using language of force, and we can slow the whole practice down. Follow the guidelines to offer accessible classes, because they will also help reduce the likelihood of injury.

However, sometimes compensation needs to be allowed (to a degree). For example, in Tabletop position, if you pick up one leg and start doing knee circles to work on hip mobility, most people will then lean off to the opposite side. You may think that means you need to address core stabilization and bringing the spine back to center to encourage engagement around the moving hip—which is right—but students could also be leaning off to the side because the *wrist* on the side with the lifted leg cannot bear that much weight for that long. If you insist on them being even, you could encourage injurious wrist compression.

The hope is that they develop an overall movement practice that can accommodate hands-and-knees work, but that you as a facilitator also understand that change takes time. You cannot necessarily move someone from a "wrong" alignment to a "right" alignment and be completely safe and effective.

Unless you are a movement expert who can look at the holistic patterns of movement and interpret what you are looking at, we should refer students with injuries and severe concerns to someone who can. Once they have a program to address some of the possibly troublesome areas, they have their homework and their yoga classes to do!

Generally speaking, yoga teachers should be recommending a diversity of movement and movement practices that mobilize across all joints frequently. The best way to prevent injury is to load your muscles and connective tissues progressively and use a diversity of approaches to movement.

Boundaries Reduce Compensation

Once you can better predict common compensation techniques, it is easier to see how boundaries encourage better movement and help us improve the efficiency of exercises. Setting boundaries begins with strong foundations—let us see why.

Stability, defined earlier as the ability to prevent movement, is necessary to channel muscular force into desired areas of the body. Think of a high lunge posture in which the student dramatically sways their lower back—we may invite them to bend their back knee, draw their navel in, lengthen the sides of their hips, etc. These cues are all in an effort to properly engage the core muscles in order to stabilize the lower back, preventing unwanted movement there, and redistributing the engagement of the posture across the body.

This is trickier when the foundation is unstable, including when standing, and the lack of boundaries allows for more unwanted movement and possibly less specific engagement. There is a popular quote from Canadian strength coach Charles

Poliquin: "You can't shoot a cannon out of a canoe." There has to be sufficient stability with a good foundation for movement before introducing specificity in movement. Because a canoe wobbles with the movement of water, the cannonball is not going to go very far, or the canoe may even move backward.

Stability is not rigidity; it includes being able to make conscious choices in movement. Referring back to our high lunge example, if you were to ask a room full of people to simply go from a high lunge to lying on the ground without any more instruction than that, you would see only unique ways of getting there. Ask them to do it multiple times and the movement would follow a different path every time—even if it looked *mostly* the same, it would *still* vary along the path to some degree.

There is a lot of value in this kind of practice—the fluidity, the reduced fear of getting a movement "right," the novelty, and problem solving for the nervous system are all great practices. Your practices should include natural movement without boundaries, but we should also learn to replicate movements and engage specifically to improve specific mobility.

To help people learn specific engagement, we have to increase the boundaries around the targeted joint. Physiologically, we are teaching people how to generate neural drive (how to "turn on" a muscle) and direct the force of contractions into specific areas (recruiting motor units) while relaxing others. When I teach, I dramatically increase the number of activities performed on the back, as well as in seated and crouching positions, because the close positioning of the body relevant to the ground provides stronger boundaries than standing postures.

Standing up provides many movement patterns that have their place in practice, but working closer to the floor only provides a few, so students can strengthen more specifically. This is the inspiration for many functional movement activities—strong boundaries to effectively direct effort.

Joint Whack-a-Mole

Before we move on from compensation, this is a cute way of thinking about how unconsciously students try to "do the thing."

Postures reveal the law of compensation: People will unconsciously make the pose happen by exploiting flexibility in other joints, even if they are not a flexible body generally. A common sight is a high lunge where teachers insist that the lunging leg's knee be stacked over the ankle while also promoting the depth of the lunge (getting lower).

I call this kind of compensation "joint whack-a-mole," inspired by the carnival game. If you force one joint into your vision of ideal alignment, another may pop out of alignment elsewhere. Poses and movements make complex requests of bodies; the ability to execute them depends on physiology, body awareness, and habitual movement patterns. Unless you have significant experience and training, it is hard to know precisely why someone is compensating.

Another example: If you imagine you are in Tabletop position, elevate your right leg straight behind you, and then bend your right knee up toward your right shoulder. If you realistically imagine yourself doing this pose, you would probably admit that you would lean to the left. Now, some leaning to the left is fine, even when there is strong mobility present, but many people lean *dramatically* to the left because it is the only way they can achieve this steep hip/knee flexion and core strength move.

To help people engage the right musculature at the right time, you want to encourage them to keep their spines at center and lean to the opposite side less by drawing their lower belly in and squeezing their gluteal muscles.

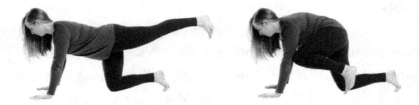

The exercise known as bird dogs typically allows the spine to move – up, down, and away from the moving leg. We can better develop the muscles of the lifted leg's hip by reducing movement in the spine.

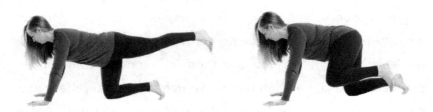

This picture reminds us that stopping short of shoulder does not mean there is less benefit in the exercise, but that the participant is successfully stabilizing their torso to prevent leaning to one side.

What Makes Good Movement

IF LESS SKILLFUL MOVEMENT can look awkward or like some joints are not particularly cooperating, what does good movement look like? Good movement is like charisma—it can be hard to define, but you know it when you see it. Coordination is a harmonious interaction of all the joints of the body, where muscles and joints cooperate as a team to achieve a requested goal.

Good movement is not necessarily about vast ranges of movement, but more about how you use it. A dancer may have a massive range of movement and use that to perform their dance, but that same range could be wearing down the cartilage in the hip socket and eventually cause a labral tear (damage to the labrum, a ring of cartilage surrounding the hip joint).

Good movement is about having options and being able to make choices—being able to choose to move or not move (stability), and to perform a precise movement as well as bear a load (strength).

When we learn a movement with competency, we stop attending to sensory input. The sensory feedback still exists, but our brain does not use it once the motor pattern is established. When the performer is doing a perfected activity, even aberrant sensory input can be added and the movement continues.

During the learning phase, sensory input is used—that is why learning movements can look awkward and shaky—but eventually movements smooth out as we learn through trial and error what information is useful. We eventually stop attending to anything that is not directly useful for the performance, which may be why some people see yoga as a moving meditation.

Dr. Eric Cobb, a chiropractor in Arizona, says we can identify skillful movement by looking for "arches not angles." Sharp angles followed by flat lines indicate a disjointed approach to movement, rather than the fluid arch of center-to-periphery skilled movement.

The way I think of this most clearly in a yoga context is when a student lifts an arm in a classical standing yoga twist, like a wide-legged twist (*Parivrtta Prasarita Padottanasana*). Often they can adopt the foundation, position their grounded hand, and lift their opposite arm, but their wrist and hand may rotate in the opposite direction they are trying to position, creating a sharp, odd angle in the wrist.

Your yoga practice should provide diversity to your daily movements. You can teach poses in different ways to illuminate what they offer, such as our more upright Chair pose (*Utkatasana)* with downward heel pressure. However, you can also forego poses altogether and use practical, unfamiliar activities—like adding movement to otherwise static postures. That movement can be specific, like holding a block to lift and lower, and it can also be exploratory and organic. Simply swaying, side bending, flexing and extending, shifting balance, etc.—these are all powerful ways to explore postures.

Not sure where to begin? Simply start to move in your practice. Try introducing little movements and "add on" changes, and enjoy the exploration and honing of your movement intuition.

While articulating good movement can be difficult, we know it when we see it. You can look at a picture of an elite athlete or dancer and recognize that their movement is skillful, even in stillness.

As yoga teachers, our job includes finding creative ways to express the components of good movement to our students. This is not necessarily metaphorical, though it can be, but when you learn a dry-yet-effective descriptor of movement, make it a part of your regular cueing practice.

Body Maps

Earlier in the book we looked at motor units—the bundles of muscle fibers (cells) that are innervated by a neuron of the nervous system. We considered how the nervous system communicates with the body, but is there a lasting impact on the brain?

The key to understanding body awareness (proprioception) and good movement is a discovery of modern neuroscience: body maps. Body maps are networks in the brain that interpret signals and direct movement for different regions of the body. Each region has a dedicated network responsible for moving and sensing that part of the body. When you consciously move a specific part of your body, you strengthen its body map in the brain[36]. Strengthened body maps make for easily accessible movement patterns; this is why so much of your movement feels effortlessly automatic.

Again, this is a demonstration of your indivisible body-mind—if the part of your brain controlling your index finger were stimulated, you would move your index finger, and when your index finger is touched, this part of your brain is active.

As we discussed in the introduction to The Bodymind, your body has different types of receptors throughout the system that feed information to the brain. Sensory receptors send information about pressure, like touch, and temperature. Other specialized receptors send information about muscle contractions and movement.

When these receptors sense a mechanical force, the nervous system conveys that message to the corresponding region of the brain. The brain interprets the signals to create a sense of where various parts of the body are in space[37].

This is a self-perpetuating cycle: We develop movement patterns because we use them as dictated by the brain, but they also shape our maps because we use them (*samskaras*).

People lean into developed body maps—when they can pull or push things with their hands, which have robust body maps, they will. They will tense their faces, do strange things with their tongues and jaws, all in an effort to execute movements that do not involve them. Learning to move well means learning to relax the face and use nominal influence of hands so that the rest of our body maps develop and we create strength/stability in the lesser developed regions of the body.

Motor Cortical Homunculus

A way to visually represent body maps is the "motor cortical homunculus." The word "homunculus" comes from the Latin word that translates to "little man."

The motor cortical homunculus visually represents the discrepancy between body part size and the number of receptors in that area. Areas of the body that look large and powerful to

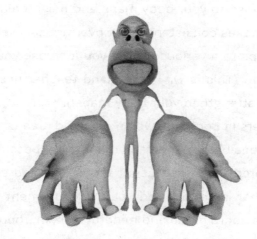

A cortical homunculus visually represents the proportion of your brain's neurons in terms of how they are dedicated to particular body parts. The size of the hands and tongue on this model may help explain why you clench these parts of your body through tricky ranges of movement.

our perception are not mapped with the level of detail given to smaller regions responsible for precise movement. With their incredible nuance and skillfulness, the hands, lips, and face occupy vast swaths of the brain (motor cortex, specifically). Their fine movements require ample mapping, where the legs' powerful muscles may be able to bear higher loads but are comparatively uncomplicated in their movement patterns.

Based on my observations, this is one of the reasons yoga students get terribly enthusiastic with any posture where they can hold onto something: when they have a toe, foot, or bind... they pull. The pulling is the movement that makes the most sense to their body maps to achieve what they think is the optimal posture (yet another reason to demonstrate and encourage moderation!).

Mapping Movement

Creating change to your body maps and heightening your proprioception takes consistent effort over time. As you strengthen body maps to a various region, you increase your precision in movement. (This is why your piano teacher needed you to practice, to strengthen your body maps!).

Taxi drivers in London have an enlarged area of their cortex that is responsible for geographic mapping, because they access that information and use it repeatedly and consistently. Similarly, when a certain body part or movement is used repeatedly in a coordinated and mindful fashion, there are actual physical and observable changes in the part of the brain that controls that body part or movement. This is part of the reason why you get better at what you practice.

Of course, not all movements are created equal in their ability to stimulate the body maps. Passive stretching does not technically improve body maps, even if it has other benefits. When your movement practice is diverse, balances both repetition and novelty, varies the sensory input (texture, surfaces, body positioning, etc), and prioritizes mindfulness, you will see change.

Changes can happen quite quickly—there is evidence that practicing reading Braille will change the brain temporarily in just four days,[38] but you would have to keep up this effort over a long period of time to effect more permanent changes.

As stressed throughout the book, we can create a plan for repetition and skill refinement, but also diversity. Strike a balance between creating some movement goals, as well as mobilizing and connecting, calming, and grounding across your whole self.

Which Muscles When

Another characteristic of good movement is using the right musculature for the right task. Generally speaking, there are three types of muscles we consider in movement.

Prime mover: contracts to create the movement

Stabilizer: contracts to prevent unwanted movement

Antagonist muscle: relaxes to allow movement (reflex)

The agonist/antagonist debate is pretty much put to rest—it is not true that *only* one muscle engages and the others relax to allow for movement. Still, there is a reflex (an automatic electrical impulse) that relaxes some musculature temporarily to allow for action elsewhere. Your muscle cannot completely relax, because if, for example, your tricep *completely* relaxed while you contracted your bicep, your fist would fling into your shoulder...or face!

The concept of prime movers and stabilizers is helpful because good movement should produce force in the right places. Big, strong muscles should be big and robust to provide stability, while smaller muscles are better for coordination.

Some of the biggest muscles are near the middle of the body: the gluteal group, abdominal muscles, hamstrings, quadriceps, hip flexors, and spinal erectors. Each of these plays a substantial role in the movement of the pelvis, which is the largest bony mass of the body (even though femurs usually get called out as the biggest single bone, the pelvis is more complicated in its movement).

Muscles of the forearms and hands, ankles, and feet are smaller, and excellent at precise movements such as writing, playing the piano and typing, kicking a ball, throwing a punch, or giving a high five.

For many yoga practitioners, if the big, stabilizing muscles of the body are insufficiently strong, the small muscles of the hands and feet will do the stabilizing work, causing these muscles to fatigue or receive overly compressive loads. So, in some ways, to strengthen the core, hips, and legs is to strengthen the wrist as well.

As yoga teachers, it is your job to help people find ways to recruit musculature and proper engagement through effective cueing and education so that they strengthen these large muscles and reduce strain on smaller ones.

Tension and Contractions

Muscle contraction is the activation of motor units, sometimes referred to as "tension generating sites" when talking about movement physiology. In movement terms, muscle contraction does not necessarily mean muscle shortening, because muscle tension can be produced without changes in muscle length, such as holding something heavy but remaining still. When you stop contracting a muscle, the muscle fibers relax to a low tension-generating state.

Muscle contractions can be described based on two variables: length and tension. There are a few different ways that a muscle can generate force relevant to the practice of yoga.

Concentric Contractions—Muscle Actively Shortening

When a muscle is activated to lift a load, it begins to shorten. Contractions that permit the muscle to shorten are referred to as concentric contractions (example: a concentric contraction is in the raising of a weight during a bicep curl).

In concentric contractions, the force generated by the muscle is always less than the muscle's maximum. These are the types of movements that generally generate muscle mass, like repetitions at the gym.

Eccentric Contractions—Muscle Actively Lengthening

During normal activity, muscles are often active while they are lengthening. A classic example is setting an object down gently (the elbow flexors must be active to control the fall of the object).

As the load on the muscle increases, a point is reached where the external force on the muscle is greater than the force that the muscle can generate. So even though the muscle may be fully activated, it is forced to lengthen due to the high external load. This is referred to as an eccentric contraction.

There are two main things to note here. First, the muscular tension achieved is higher than the muscle's ability to generate force, so you can set down a much heavier object than you can lift. Second, the ability to generate tension is not hugely dependent on length, which suggests that skeletal muscles (big muscles close to the bones) are very resistant to lengthening. We do know that the further a joint moves into extension, away from a neutral place, the less safe it is, so we do not generally train at the extreme end of our ranges of movement.

There is a lot of exciting research into using eccentric contractions as more efficient methods of strengthening.

Eccentric and concentric contractions are typically the contractions that take us *into* and *out of* yoga postures, so when we add movement to postures or integrate functional movement exercises, we are employing these contractions.

Isometric Contraction—Muscle Actively Held at a Fixed Length

A third type of muscle contraction, isometric contraction, is one in which the muscle is activated, but instead of being allowed to lengthen or shorten, it is held at a constant length. An example of an isometric contraction would be carrying a cork block between extended hands. The weight of the block would pull downward with gravity, but your hands and arms would be opposing the motion with equal force pressing upward. Since your arms are neither raising nor lowering, your biceps will be isometrically contracting.

Integrating Motor Learning Theories into Yoga Classes

Bridging the bodymind and movement principles, let us revisit motor learning principles and specifically connect them to teaching yoga before we move on to the "Accessible Yoga" section.

Change happens in stages.

Thoughtfully designed yoga practices balance short-term satisfaction with long-term gains. You meet today's needs of some exercise and some stretching, while also including techniques like *pranayama*, taking care of more vulnerable joints, and less "feelings-intensive" movement practices.

Talk to your students about the different aspects of practice, including reminders that an activity does not need to produce a specific feeling of stretch or strength to be beneficial.

Encouraging students to relax their "maximum utility" mindset of yoga makes for a non-competitive atmosphere.

Sharing stories of what yoga means to you and your skill development across yoga's limbs will remind students that it is okay to be who they are, where they are, while reminding you of that fact too.

Variable practice is essential, a sort of "repetition without repetition," so there are variations of the same movement.

Take multiple approaches to *yoga-asana*, including sometimes focusing on alignment and nuance, and sometimes focusing on just getting yourself moving and enjoying that movement. Different approaches to practice are all welcome.

My favorite example is Goddess pose *(Utkata Konasana)*! When reviewing this list, remember that variation can include positioning, tempo, props, etc. You can:

* Hold Goddess pose like classical *asana* and experiment with isometric contractions and endurance
* Add a block to be squeeze, or exercise bands held under the feet and stretched upward by the hands
* Add a mudra or change your arm position
* Change your foot position or focus on toes lifting and spread or toes down and spreading
* Move into and out of the posture like a sumo squat activity at a steady pace
* Slowly "trickle" up and down, out of and into the posture to explore the interconnectedness of joints and

notice the shifting relationship between joint positions as you gradually change shape

Motor learning involves the learner in the goal setting.

We want to encourage students to learn about themselves and their embodied experiences. When we offer options and use language that sounds invitational and exploratory, we involve our students in this exploration. "You may want to..." becomes empowering and encourages students to experiment, rather than positioning teaching as a conveyance of rules.

There are many different types/approaches to practice (verbally walking through the steps of a task, doing part of the whole, doing the whole task, etc.).

Yoga offers such a wide variety of aspects of practice, including visualization, breaking down the movement, breathwork, etc., that there seems to be limitless ways to explore technique. For a more in-depth conversation on demonstrating, see that section of the book, but know that there is always a place for different approaches.

Provide the learner with feedback so that they can recognize their intuitive feedback of what "feels right."

Watch your classes move so that you can encourage them when they are moving well and responding to your feedback. Share with them what something may feel like or what it may not feel like, always with the caveat that individuals feel differently, and feelings of the body should be honed and listened to over time. Say less about where stretch should occur, and instead diversify your understanding of how people experience yoga, so your cueing is invitational and less prescriptive. Encourage your students to place their attention (focus of their mind) holistically or specifically, but not necessarily in search of feeling.

PART FOUR

Principles of
Accessible Yoga

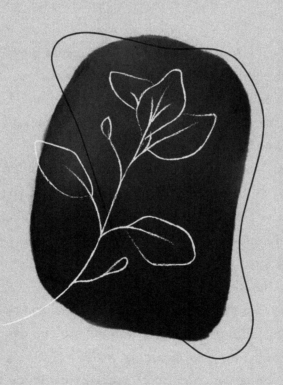

Accessible Yoga

WHAT MAKES YOGA ACCESSIBLE or inaccessible? The term implies that people can "access" it, which assumes there are no financial, cultural, linguistic, or mobility barriers. To address all of these barriers, I know many social justice activists and politicians who would love some advice.

I feel that this raises a meaningful conversation and an opportunity for yoga teachers to remember that yoga studio classes will not be accessible to everyone. Teaching yoga to specific populations is often most successful when offered in spaces they already gather and live in, and many of the principles here will still help you in your teaching.

To convey that studios are inclusive spaces, and not just for young, skinny, and mobile white women, studios can improve their visual marketing by including yogis of a variety of ages, ethnicities, mobilities, and body shapes. To reduce financial barriers, some studios offer classes for reduced fees, go into the community to teach, or exchange memberships for helping around the studio.

One of the goals of this book is to improve the accessibility of group mat classes, so our definition of accessible yoga in this book refers to an *asana/pranayama*/meditation practice, where participants will have the prerequisite mobility to mostly participate. They may occasionally need the stabilizing help of a wall to balance on one foot, and they require intelligently sequenced classes (as we cover in this book), but they are capable of getting onto the ground and getting back up if you provide an unhurried pace.

If you are teaching yoga, spending time on the internet, or spending time in spaces that do not focus on accessible yoga, it is easy to get an incomplete impression of what bodies can do. For example, my teacher trainees are shocked when I tell them that the transition of Three-legged Dog pose, "stepping through," and standing up into a High Lunge, is not an accessible transition. I typically hear back from them a few months after they start teaching, when they confirm that this transition is, in fact, more difficult or impossible for more people than they suspected.

The yoga landscape has changed dramatically, and this is an aspect of service where there is still work to do. Thirty years ago, when yoga was more of a fringe practice in the West, it was likely that many yoga practitioners saw headstands and Wheel *(Chakrasana)* and Crow poses *(Bakasana)* as desirable goals of the practice. If not those, they had some idea of their practice advancing through posture performance.

As yoga becomes popularized as a wellness practice, more and more people are practicing to *maintain* their range of movement, manage their stress, and improve their overall health. However, as terrific as weekly yoga is (I am a cheerleader for all who practice once a week!), it can only do so much. If someone is beginning a yoga practice in mid-life and they are practicing once a week, the input is not sufficient to create dramatic changes.

In the pressure to attract yoga customers, many studios position themselves as offering accessible or "yoga for every body" classes that still require at least an average to high level of mobility. Yoga is a tough industry, but we should still be willing to send students to other studios and teachers if we are not purposefully trying to teach more accessible classes.

Developing techniques for improving yoga accessibility may come more quickly if we first identify what makes yoga classes inaccessible. We will begin with the most obvious and move to the more atmospheric.

Identifying Tricky Activities

Tricky Postures and Prerequisite Mobility

Activities that have highly specific prerequisite mobility will not be accessible to the general population. Elsewhere in this book I talk about how to offer trickier postures in an accessible yoga class so that everyone has a meaningful experience. But first, let's consider "trickiness" in yoga and explore the idea of pre-requisite mobility—the requirement for pre-existing strength and flexibility to be able to participate in some *asana* activities.

First, consider the "classical" transition from Plank pose (*Phalakasana*) into Upward-facing Dog (*Urdhva Mukha Svanasana*).

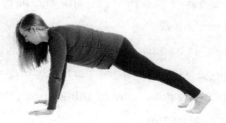

* Requires sufficient strength in the trunk, shoulders, and legs to reduce excessive compression in wrists
* Requires sufficient wrist flexibility to allow for steep angle and high load
* Requires flexibility in the feet and toes sufficient to steeply flex the "curled under toes" of Plank pose

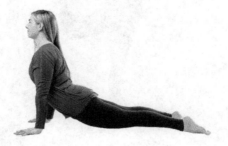

Similarly, Upward-facing Dog requires high levels of ankle flexibility in the plantar flexion direction. If someone cannot extend their ankle in that position, bear weight on their ankles and hands, attain the flexibility for the big backbend, and summon the strength to keep their legs off the ground, they cannot do this posture.

This is how we can think about the potential for doing a yoga posture—what is the prerequisite mobility (strength and flexibility) and stability?

It is not a perfect analysis, since some activities could develop these things without having perfectly desirable ranges of movement, but it is a good way to think about the less obvious challenges of *yoga-asana*.

We can also consider Dancer's pose (*Natarajasana*), for example.

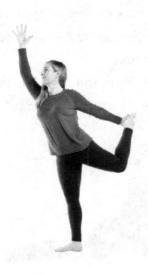

♦ Requires sufficient stability to stand on one foot and balance, and the ability to bend a knee deeply enough to catch hold of the foot

- Requires body awareness to help student find their other foot without necessarily seeing it, and requires the strength to hold their leg
- Requires flexibility in shoulder extension to reach behind, hold a foot, and allow the arm to be held straight in traction
- Requires hip flexibility for extension initially, and then possibly into flexion depending on the version

Whenever I ask teacher trainee groups to describe the prerequisite mobility of a balance posture, it never occurs to them that the first one is to be able to *stand on one foot*. The stability required to stand on one foot is a great gift—yogis and therapists who specialize in yoga for seniors and fall prevention know that whether or not a person can balance on one foot is an excellent predictor of the risk of a future fall. Falls can be devastating for seniors, so any yoga program that promotes longevity should be emphasizing safely balancing on one foot as a component of that.

That means that if we ever teach a balance posture with some flexibility/strength requirements to it, we should be working one foot. You can share that with your students, and then they can practice simply lifting a heel off the ground to disrupt balance enough to build stability.

There is tremendous value to simply standing on one foot. Dancer's pose has some backbend and unilateral hip extension—you can achieve these movements with a Camel pose (*Ustrasana*) variation and a Low Lunge (*Anjaneyasana*).

You may be thinking, *In considering prerequisite mobility, does that mean I have to ensure all students are very properly aligned?*

Nope! As we discussed in the section on compensation and "joint whack-a-mole," you cannot force one joint into "ideal alignment" without the body compensating elsewhere. If we offer activities that are in generally accessible positions and where the load is evenly distributed around the working joints, we do not need to worry so much about whether their shape looks ideal. Bodies are resilient when programming is sensible.

Tricky Transitions

Hopefully you now understand that postures have prerequisite mobility—some muscles have to be able to relax, some joints have to be able to bear a load at a particular angle, etc. Transitions are the same. If you look between two postures, you can see all kinds of required mobility needed to transition between them. For example, in my younger days, I enjoyed teaching Chair pose *(Utkatasana)* into Crow pose *(Bakasana)*. What does it require?

- ◆ The mobility to first achieve Chair pose, which typically includes hip flexion and shoulder flexion by lifting your arms
- ◆ The stability to balance as both heels lift *and* as you begin to descend toward the ground (this is advanced balance)

- The ability to bear weight on your toe joints—as you descend toward the ground, your whole body weight is bearing on extremely extended toe joints
- The ability to sustain deeply flexed hips in order to get your knees onto your arms (and sustain your body weight on your arms via your knees), in addition to holding steeply flexed knees as you move onto your hands
- The ability to steeply flex your wrists to perform Crow and all of its mobility/stability requirements

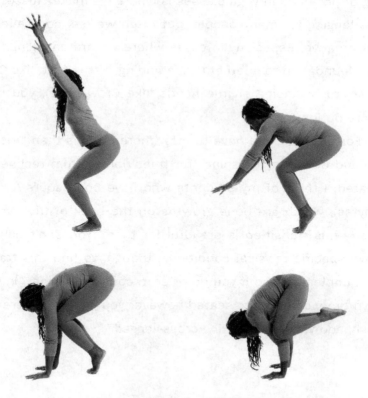

This sequence shows the transition from Chair (*Utkatasana*) to Crow pose (*Bakasana*)

For younger, more mobile yogis, these challenging transitions can feel fun, invigorating, and captivating, since they demand so much of your attention. However, when you break down the transitions and see what they require, you can quickly see how many people would be left out if you were to include this in an average-mobility class.

Part of the reason I likely enjoyed this transition so much is because it was sequenced toward the middle and end of classes, and then we could go from Crow pose to a seated position (also easy for mobile bodies). Not considering the changing of positions in yoga classes is where we make classes too challenging for many people, but often we feel compelled to get creative. Especially in cases where we are changing from one foundation to another (i.e., standing on the feet, like Chair pose, to balancing on the hands, like Crow pose), you need more options.

For example, you *have* to offer more options than "rocking up and down on the spine" for transitioning from reclined to seated. I think of my students who have bone spurs (osteophytes), which are bone growths on the back of their vertebrae—this transition is dreadful for them. You don't have to have specific physical conditions, though, to find this transition unpleasant, so if you do offer it, consider saying, "In your own time, come up to seated however you want to. There's no rush, and we'll meet sitting cross-legged."

If you prefer specific suggestions, you could offer these three:

1. Roll onto one side and press your way to seated.
2. Rocking along the length of the spine until you come to seated.
3. DIY! However you want to come to seated, let's meet there...

Overloading Specific Joints

Everyone has had a moment in a yoga class where they wished a sequence would move on from one position because something is aching, and some areas are more prone to this than others.

Let's look at three areas I feel are most likely to cause pain or discomfort in prolonged sequences, beginning with the wrists.

Wrists

Even though the small musculature of the hands and wrists *can* be trained to take body weight in advanced postures like handstands, it can take years to safely train for these positions.

Even in hands-and-knees positions, there is still a lot of pressure on the wrists in a flexed position.

Plank *(Phalaksana)*, Downward-facing Dog *(Adho Mukha Svanasana)*, and Tabletop poses all create situations where the wrists can be leaned into too much. Here are a few ways to alleviate wrist compression:

♦ Roll up the front end of the mat to elevate wrists into a lesser degree of flexion

- Use a yoga wedge (a thin, triangular prop used to elevate the heel of the hand) to do the same
- If the student's hand can fit, placing their palms on a block with their fingers over the edge also seems to help, especially for pregnant students, because it removes full extension of the palm but also shifts their center of gravity
- Position fists knuckles-down, with fingers pointing inward (this is also a great position for strengthening, so you may want to include this as a component of the activity, rather than just as a modification)
- Alternate between palms down and tented fingers, which strengthens the hand/wrist muscles and relies less on flexibility
- Alternate between Tabletop (arms extended) and forearms down for poses like Dolphin *(Ardha Pincha Mayurasana)* and mobility activities using Dolphin
- Place blocks underneath forearms
- Walk the hands forward to reduce the angle of wrist flexion

Knees

It is not just aging or lower-mobility students who will spend time in Tabletop pose—it is a pose that pregnant students will spend time in too, since laying on their front can be uncomfortable and even nausea-inducing. Wrists aren't the only joints that suffer from prolonged compression here—many people will struggle with pressure on their knees. Here are a few ways we can alleviate knee pressure.

- Encourage students to place a folded blanket mid-way up their mats for knee padding, and build a sequence that ensures the blanket will not be interfered with so it can stay where it is
- Make silicone knee-jellies a props purchase for your classes, since they're lightweight, easy to wash, and are easy to tote around
- Alternate between activities that have both knees down in Tabletop and postures that take the pressure off at least one knee, like walking hands back toward your legs and lifting up into Gate pose *(Parighasana)* variations
- Alternate between activities that have both knees down and prone postures (lying on the belly) to do some back strengthening, like lifting in and out of Locust posture
- Use Tabletop posture activities to replace the Plank pose *(Phalakasana)* and lower backbend sequence of Sun Salutations, so the work gets done but you move on after a few minutes

Lunge-heavy Classes

When the students in the room cannot do shoulder-intensive strengthening movements from classical *yoga-asana*, teachers may unconsciously pack the strengthening elements of class with Warrior postures and a variety of lunges, including side lunges.

Your legs have bigger muscles that can bear heavier loads, and these muscles have less variety of positioning as the shoulders, so there is a lower likelihood of acute injuries. Remember that we want to evenly distribute force across the body, so consider the following options.

- Learn shoulder strengthening exercises that focus more on mobility than strength to integrate into class in typical yoga foundations (reclined, seated, etc.)
- Include functional movement exercises, like scapular push-ups, for classes with average to higher levels of mobility
- Try integrating little weights, weighted balls, or resistance bands to add load and increase resistance in a variety of foundations for classes with lower to average mobility levels
- Diversify your leg exercises, including side-lying leg strengthening, so that you are mobilizing around the whole hip and leg area

Accessible Atmosphere

The tangible ways that yoga is inaccessible to many participants are further entrenched by the more cultural and atmospheric ways that yoga is inaccessible. Initially we talked about some of the financial and cultural barriers to practice, but there are also in-class approaches that are very much within the teacher's control to promote accessible yoga.

Non-Competitive Class Culture

Competition is a part of human nature and life, but it does not need to be a part of the yoga culture—this is a practice that promotes union, not differentiation.

We may feel less competitive with others and ourselves when the environment is friendly and convivial. Getting to know students and making an effort to include other students in conversations promotes a welcoming atmosphere. New students can find it especially hard to walk into a new yoga space. It's important to make yourself available and open for conversation.

Arrive early enough to your classes that you can greet people, and when opportunity arises, get to know your students. Occasionally, I sit down on someone's mat to say, "You know Leslie, I know you love hip mobility activities, but I have no idea what you do outside the yoga room."

As facilitators, we also want to balance encouragement for students in practice, while at the same time, acknowledging yoga should not include feelings of desperation or endurance-at-all-costs—taking breaks is a self-compassion practice.

Changing the Goals of Yoga

Yes, setting goals is a great way to provide direction for our spirit and energy, and there is evidence that goal setting is conducive to cultivating a positive outlook. What implicitly happens when teachers talk about "the goal of this posture" is that *you* end up setting goals for students, rather than encouraging them to set goals and intentions for themselves.

We may unconsciously cultivate a competitive, goal-oriented culture of yoga when we talk about how "eventually" the pose will do such and such a thing, or the "advanced version" will achieve X, Y, or Z.

It may be true that doing a handstand will cultivate a sense of adventure and curiosity, "change our perspective," or offer the benefits of strong balance and shoulder and core strength. However, it is just as true that some people are proportionately and physically predisposed to performing handstands more easily, and that predisposition can be used to cultivate strong attachments to ego as much as curiosity.

When you talk about intention and goal setting with your students, encourage them to see self-compassion and compassion for others, living with less pain, mental calm, good sleep, and fortitude as the goals of practice.

Common Embodiment: The General Population

As this book emphasizes, diverse movement practices are good for our bodyminds. They will adapt to the loads placed on them and, without optimal engagement and activity around the joints, they eventually succumb to gravity and compensation. Over time, people rely more on the support of the fibrous connective tissues (ligaments, tendons, fascia) and the "wrong" muscles to carry out the function intended for other surrounding musculature (as we discussed in the "Compensation" section). For example, lower back muscles may work harder to replace an absence of strength/engagement in the abdominal or gluteal muscles, resulting in the feeling of tightness in the lower back.

When I say "common embodiment," I am referring to how people are showing up on yoga mats in studios and places of practice, and what their challenges could be. The following common challenges are based on observations made over years of teaching yoga to the general population and tailoring practices to manage these realities.

Head and Neck

- Tension around the eye sockets, eyebrows, cheeks, and jaw (which can cause students to struggle to relax during activities they find challenging, which varies from person to person)
- Tight neck muscles from a jutted-forward head posture (including upper trapezius and levator scapula)
- Weak neck flexors that bring the chin toward the chest (found at the front of your neck, including the sternocleidomastoid, the big muscle you can see and feel on the side of your neck that starts under your ear and runs to your clavicle)
- Tight neck extensors (limiting any "looking up" movement)

Trunk and Arms

- Tight chest muscles (pectorals) and fronts of the shoulders (anterior deltoids) from a rounded chest

- Weak mid-back with a limited ability to extend the spine in this area (mid-trapezius and lower trapezius, rhomboids, and serratus anterior)
- Weak thoracic spine (upper back, including upper trapezius, and levator scapula, which lifts the scapula)
- Weak wrists that limit the amount of time that can be spent putting pressure on them (tight/strong wrist extensors and weak/unstable wrist flexors)
- Sore lower back (due to overcompensation for weak abdominal muscles and gluteal group, absorbed pressure from pelvic tilt, and/or partially due to passive shortening of psoas/hip flexor muscles)
- Weak diaphragm that limits us to shallow breathing and feelings of insufficiently deep breaths in)

Hips and Legs

- Weak hips (three gluteus muscles) and backs of legs (hamstrings), increasing risk of shearing on lumbar vertebrae and tightness in lower back
- Tight/over-strengthened quadriceps
- Tight/strong calf muscles (gastrocnemius and soleus)
- Weak feet causing limited ankle stability/mobility

That is a long list of potential muscle ailments, but it is a list that *really matters* to how we sequence and develop our yoga classes.

To maximize the efficiency of the practice, especially for students who only practice once a week, we need to creatively sequence in ways that strengthen and mobilize thoroughly, without placing undue strain on another part of the body.

Journaling Activity

• •

How do you strike a balance between providing classes that help people improve their mobility while also working with their current embodiment?

What have your experiences of "tightness" and limitations been like? How have they changed in relationship to your lifestyle, age, and movement practices?

Evolving, Not Replacing, Yoga-Asana

To meet the needs of the average person and explore what is beneficial and healthful for bodyminds, yoga teachers are exploring many movement modalities and how to integrate them into yoga classes.

Now that we have a list of muscles commonly lacking development that we may need to address in a yoga practice, our sequences should provide some needed movement. Many practitioners fail to engage specific muscles, and instead lean into where they can already move. To increase body awareness and sound control, we have to actively engage muscles we may not be accustomed to engaging, rather than only using habitual movement patterns.

Unfortunately, many poses are inefficient at encouraging the use of underdeveloped muscles, and the goal of building body awareness between poses can get lost. For example, Chair pose (*Utkatasana*) has the potential to produce better strength in the hamstrings, improve balance, and even build better oblique abdominal strength—it is better practiced more upright than it typically is, and with downward pressure through the heels. Most of us have stronger muscles on the front of our legs (in the quadriceps group) than the back of our legs, so yogis tend to sit low and pitch their torsos forward, which strengthens already-strong muscles. We can do it this way, and we should try changing the approach, too, and explore all variations.

We do not need to eliminate "classical" yoga postures from our classes because they offer their value in endurance, steadfastness, exploration, and experience of subtle energy (*prana*). I find the greatest calm and clarity in static postures. However, I recommend weaving other movement activities between yoga postures, so students get the benefit of targeted, specific effort of both rolling-around-on-the-ground playfulness, and the observational quality of yoga postures. Movement activities also provide excellent warm-ups for more static practices.

What Is Functional Movement?

Functional movement is a term that emerged from physiotherapy screening to help identify dysfunctional movement patterns in clients. The development of courses of treatment in physiotherapy has a similar history to yoga and other movement practices and therapy modalities in terms of addressing pain, injury, and limitation—address the issue locally, rather than looking at the body as a whole.

If you have a hip complaint, you possibly attack that area with stretching, foam rolling, and topical analgesics. We now realize that movement in the body is a coordinated effort that can be localized to highly specific levels, but across the spectrum, the whole body is participating.

Functional movement screening involves a qualified professional evaluating a person's ability to perform fundamental movements and identifying areas of weakness, inhibition, and dysfunction. Based on the assessment, they can then recommend exercises that address the whole.

The body is interconnected and complicated enough that shoulder complaints can arise from pelvic floor dysfunction! As a new yoga teacher, that can feel intimidating, but I have a suggestion to ease the fear: simply teach well-rounded classes that promote a diversity of movements and activities.

Functional movement exercises have come to mean any exercise that promotes good movement and joint functionality, but I like adding that they also help us live independently and with ease.

It is a functional movement to be able to lift your arms over your head as you age so you can reach shelves, or to roll your body out of your bed. These are simple but profound needs that can be addressed through yoga practice.

There is an intelligent design that underpins your physiology, and that physiology requires maintenance in order to provide you with a sense of stability and ease. Your muscles may be responsible for stabilizing a joint and executing a range of movements, but if they're never asked to do so, they will conform to the limited requests made of them. For example, if you only ask them to help you sit, they'll get really good at sitting.

Think of how easily many people can sit passively with their spine upright, knees bent at a 90° angle, and ankles underneath the knees. Now, try replicating that form in Chair pose (*Utkatasana*)! Part of the reason you likely can't is due to the weakness that develops from excessive sitting in that shape. The chair you sit in holds you in the shape (instead of your muscles), and the deeper layers of abdominal muscle, hip flexors, gluteal group, hamstrings, etc. all weaken from disuse.

We Shape Ourselves Through Daily Ritual

Functional movement exercises develop controlled range of movement in underused muscles so that other muscle groups don't have to compensate. In this way, they are corrective exercises that also show you how much or how little control you actually have over different parts of your body. My favorite way to demonstrate this is with your toes, because most of us are much more flexible in our feet than we are mobile—we can move our toes but can't completely control that movement. While you could learn to move each of your toes individually, which would demonstrate mobility, just curling your toes under in a kneeling position and stretching them is flexibility.

This is both an experiment and an exercise! Stand with your feet apart and step your right foot forward a little. Put your hands on your hips and look at your right foot. To build true foot strength (such a gift for a lifelong ability to balance!), press your big toe down strongly and lift and spread your other four toes. Now spread and press your four toes down strongly and lift your big toe. Repeat until you tire, noticing if your fingers and left foot are wiggling in an effort to make it happen.

Too easy? Switch to two toes down and three toes up to feel the frustration of change happening!

Teach this and other foot exercises to all your students, but particularly to those with more "chronologically experience". Even simple foot exercises promote foot mobility are positive interventions against the risk of falls as we age.

Awesome-a Exercises

The internet is full of great biotensegrity-inspired, mobility, Feldenkrais, functional movement, and targeted exercises.
To recognize the perpetual shift of trendy movement terms, but give you a few examples of what I include in class, I am calling these activities "awesome-a" to evoke the word *asana* and remind us that playfulness is part of practice.

Pencil Pickups

Get into a reclined position with one leg raised. Alternate between plantar-flexing your ankle (ballerina style) and dorsiflexing your ankle (bending it like a crouched basketball player). When you straighten your ankle, spread your toes. When you bend your ankle, curl your toes like you were trying to pick up a pencil with them.

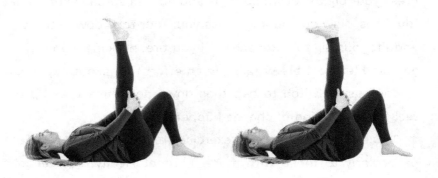

Cactus Arm Backbends

Sit with your legs extended and relaxed, and reach your arms to the ceiling and bend your elbows. Kitten paw your hands (spread your fingers and curl them a little bit) and stretch your elbows back as you lift your chest and chin, then touch your elbows toward each other in front of you and round your upper back.

As you keep repeating the movement, notice the difference between your palms coming together or your pinkies touching and palms facing you.

We keep our legs extended to keep the lower back steady—try it with legs crossed and notice how much the lower back moves instead of the desired upper back!

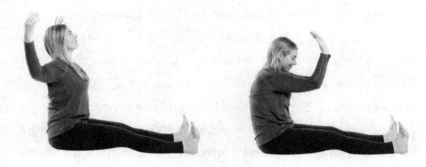

Frankenstein's Monster

Sit with your legs extended, toes pointing up to the ceiling, and arms extended straight out (parallel to your legs) in front of you like you were doing a Frankenstein's monster impression. Twist to the left while pulling your left elbow back and reaching your right arm forward. Then, do the same movement, but pulling your right elbow back. Continue to switch sides slowly. As you slowly twist back and forth, try to suck the opposite thigh bone back into its socket. Try to keep yourself erect over your pelvis, rather than leaning back.

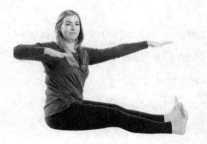 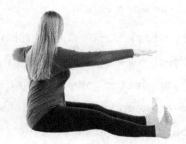

Ride a Bike, Pet the Dog

I love this activity for its endurance, creativity, and mobilizing movements. It is a space to get creative, as well as a great litmus test for a room to see how well your class moves.

From a supine (lying down) position, rock your legs over your body and start to mimic pedaling an upside-down bicycle. Dial up the pressure, so your movements are slow. Then add 15–20 inches of space between your legs, and remember—the higher your legs go, the less load there is on the lower back. Feel free to explore range. Pretend you're painting with a paintbrush held in your toes, or petting a dog with your feet. Explore side to side movement in the hips too!

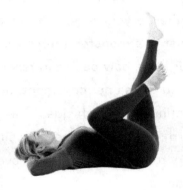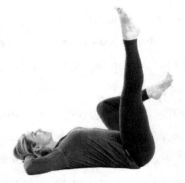

Ode to Jane Fonda

From back flat on the mat, bring legs into Butterfly pose (soles of feet together, knees open), and press down into the edges of your feet to roll your spine toward the ceiling and then back down. Keep your bum cheeks strong, try to roll up and down your spine, and barely touch the ground with your hips.

You can add pulses, and squeezing your hips toward the ceiling in a hold (it can also be nice to follow this exercise with reclined Pigeon pose, sometimes called a figure-4 stretch).

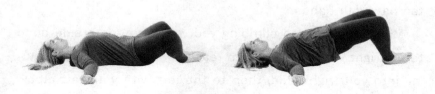

Beach Reading Hips

Lie on your left side like you were reading a book on the beach—prop your head up using your left hand. Bend your knees and pull them toward your chest, with legs stacked and your right hand on the ground in front of you. Push your feet into each other (anchoring them together) and lift them off the ground. Lift your right knee slowly, and then lower it slowly. Keep repeating this motion, while still keeping your feet pressing into each other.

If it's going well, when your knee comes up, reach forward like you were picking an apple out of a basket. As your knee comes down, pull your elbow back like you were using a bow and arrow. Keep repeating: knee up, reach forward, knee down, pull elbow back.

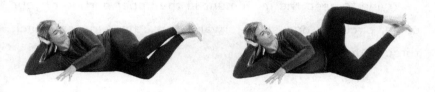

Climbing Out of a Proposal

Step into a short lunge stance—the same position you would use for a marriage proposal.

Curl your back toes under, if this is an option, and then kitten paw your hands.

Mimicking a kitten climbing your furniture, do a side bend to the right with your left arm reaching and right elbow drawing into your right side, then to the left with your left elbow drawing to your left side and right arm reaching overhead to the left.

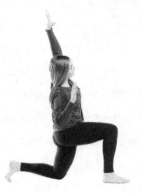 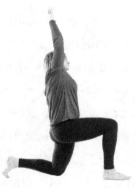

A New Wheel

Sitting cross legged, form a "square" overhead by lifting your arms and holding opposite elbows. Lift your chest, extending yourself into a backbend.

Trying to keep the movement in the upper portion of your spine, circle to one side, forward, the other side and back through the backbend.

Do a few rotations before switching your grip on your elbows and doing the other direction. Experiment with curling your fingers in and straightening them out.

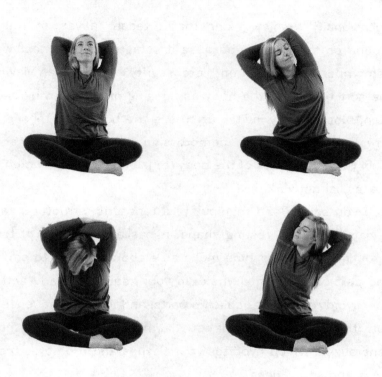

Fascia Fitness: Rolling Around on the Ground

Occasionally I enjoy joking that I teach "advanced rolling around on the ground" because it sometimes feels that way. Remember the section on biotensegrity? Rather than viewing the soft tissues of the body as hanging off the moving skeleton, biotensegrity invites us to see the body as a tensegrity structure—the skeleton (compression elements) as suspended in the soft tissues of the body (tension elements), including the fascial network.

If you squish and manipulate a tensegrity structure, as it deviates from its resting shape, it has an evenness of tone throughout it, unless you make an elaborate effort to smush one part out from the whole. In your sequencing and activities, avoid "smushing" specific parts, and instead sequence in activities of varying omnidirectional movements that are more generalized, which hydrates your tissues and promotes resilience and springiness.

When we are practicing functional movement exercises, we typically focus the effort into specific joints to train the motor units of that area to fire appropriately. In essence, there are more definite boundaries and particular efforts.

When we are rolling around on the ground, or engaging in other more organic movements that oscillate fluidly, we are supporting the tensegrity elements of our tissues—strength balanced by suppleness.

These kinds of activities, like a lot of functional movement exercises, are excellent for more than just your yogis with limited ranges of movement. They are excellent for your hyper-flexible yogis who should be learning to increase their boundaries of movement, rather than continuing to explore the end of their range of flexibility, the way a lot of *yoga-asana* inadvertently encourages.

Exercises for fascial fitness emphasize whole-body movements rather than strong boundaries; fluid, organic, sensual movements that seem to flow from one position in space to another, and focus on cultivating awareness through the journey, rather than aiming for a destination.

A Different Happy Baby

Lie on your back with bent knees. "Cactus" your arms and keep them on the ground. Bend your legs like you were going into Happy Baby, but keep your joints perky and legs separated. Rock your legs (keeping the space!) over to the right, through center, and off to the left. Rock back and forth, massaging the tissues of your low back.

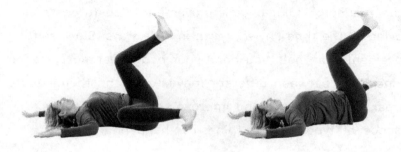

Low Back Release

Lie on your back with your knees rocked over you and your arms "cactus-ed" by your shoulders. Moderately squeeze your thighs and shins together (preventing a hamstring cramp!) and keep your heels close to your body. Tip your legs over to the right and—keeping them squeezing toward each other—separate knees and feet and bring them back together at a moderate pace. Return to center for a short break, and then switch sides.

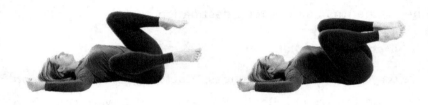

Adding Movement to Yoga Postures

As mentioned in Part Three ("Movement"), there is a lot of value in simply finding organic movement in postures. You are moving all the time anyway, even in little ways. Slow, shifting movements can help you hone your body awareness, notice connections between different movements and their effects on parts of your body, and improve stability and balance. In essence, all types of good things can happen.

You can explore this by:

* Dramatically exaggerating the slowness with which you enter and exit postures and changing elements of the pose, like adding a bent knee, or lifted arms
* Leaning side to side or forward and back, changing where you distribute your weight
* Adding movement to your pelvis or another joint
* Slow and subtle side bending back and forth, or moving forward and back and up and down

You can also add more specific movements to postures, since adding motion to a stable foundation is one of the best ways to add action to an accessible class without leaving some students behind. The activities in the previous section demonstrate many options; feel free to mix and match and see what happens when you do.

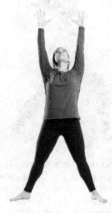
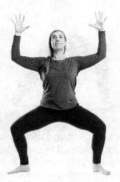

Using Goddess pose (*Utakata Konasana*) as a foundation for squats works well in many class settings. This alternative offers dynamic hip flexion and shoulder extension positions while also building heat. It is much more accessible than the similar "speed skater" movement of Side Lunge (*Skandasana*).

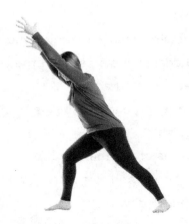
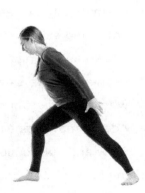

In a Warrior I foundation, which is more stable than a high lunge, you can add arm sweeps reaching forward and back. Cue the starting position as leaning forward like "someone shot you out of a cannon" or "you are flying."

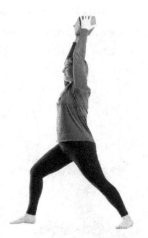
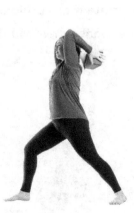

In a Warrior I foundation, you can also add shoulder mobility work when you add a block. Hold a block overhead by its short sides. Squeezing the block while you broaden across your upper back, lower the block behind your head, bending at your elbows. Encourage students to control or "hold" the space between their elbows, some people's elbows will bend out to the sides in their effort to perform the movement.

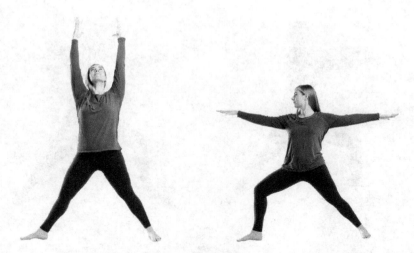

There are so many things you can do in Warrior II (*Virabhadrasana*)! Among the most simple and accessible movements is simply straightening the arms and legs to reach to the ceiling, then floating back to Warrior II slowly. Looking up and looking out over your front arm is also a healthy movement for your neck!

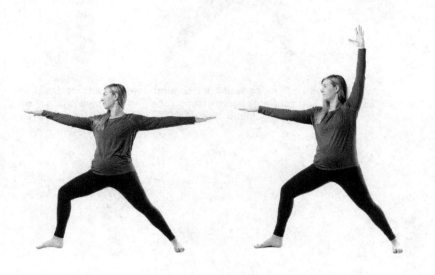

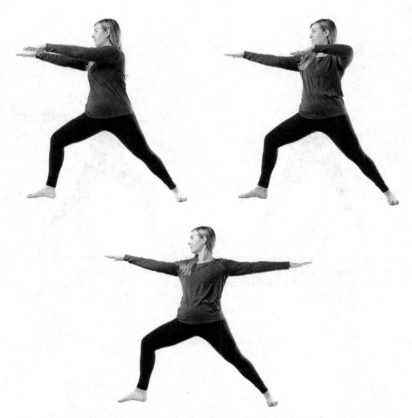

Also in Warrior II, you can swim your back arm forward like a front crawl, bend your elbow to pull your arm back, extend it behind you back to Warrior II, and repeat!

Sun Salutations: A Short History

THE SEQUENCE OF YOGA postures known as *Suryanamaskāra* (*surya* = sun, *namaskara* = salute) is a central component to most Hatha and Vinyasa practices in modern yoga. The heavy influence of Sri Pattabhi Jois's Ashtanga yoga on modern Western yoga culture and the relative accessibility and athleticism of the sequence contributed to its popularity.

Like much of *yoga-asana*, this practice likely has relatively young roots, as traced by Mark Singleton in *Yoga Body: The Origins of Modern Posture Practice*. Singleton argues that a Sun Salutation is "a mixture of yoga as medical gymnastics and body-conditioning on the one hand, and state of the art dumbbell work and freehand European bodybuilding techniques on the other."

In the early twentieth century, dynamic sequences served as warm-up exercises to prepare for various poses and weight work. Sun Salutations were not recognized, however, as part of the same body of knowledge comprising yoga before that period. Despite Jois's claims that the sequence central to

Ashtanga yoga stems from the *Vedas* (the ancient work from which Vedic sciences like yoga and Ayurveda stem), there is not much concrete evidence to this position.

Some yogis argue that the practice is more than 2,000 years old, and was part of the ritualistic greeting of the sun ingrained in Hindu religious rituals. These would have included the lighting of sacred fires, *mantra* recitation, offerings, and prostration of devotees. The rising of the sun is an auspicious time in both yoga and Ayurveda, known as *brahmamurti*, "the creator's hour."

There are many variations on the Sun Salutation, including a moon (*chandra*) version that includes a Low Lunge (*Anjaneyasana*) from Kripalu. Regardless of the practice's age, it speaks to the appealing nature of repetitive, familiar, synchronized movement.

Evolving Sun Salutations

IF YOU WANT TO teach the typical Sun Salutation and improve its accessibility, here are a couple of suggestions.

Between half lift and standing positions, insert a Chair pose (*Utkatasana*) on the way up and down.

Adding this one other familiar posture moves yogis more gradually from upright (standing at the front of the mat) to inversion (a forward fold or Downward-facing Dog). Moving this way gives more time for blood pressure to regulate, which is great for yogis who can do the physical challenges of the sequence, but whose blood pressure may not make it easy to quickly move up and down (this is true for yogis with high or low blood pressure!).

Tiptoe from Downward-facing Dog *(Adho Mukha Svanasana)* to the front of your mat, and forget about hopping or stepping.

To return from Downward-facing Dog to the front of the mat, encourage students to lift their hips and heels dramatically and tiptoe 200 tiny steps forward. Sometimes I add "like you were trying to walk into a handstand" (and one time, someone did!). Your heels will likely lower before they reach your hands, and that is okay.

This movement improves mobility by improving our ability to lengthen our spine and legs simultaneously. A student who did a four-day training session with me felt that after four days, her range of movement in terms of leg extension was better than ever before.

For mobile yogis, hopping forward may be a beneficial exercise, but this tiptoe approach makes better use of the transition than stepping forward.

Subtract the parts that are the most problematic and replace them with something more accessible.

As I emphasize in the "Sequencing" section, using one foundation for repeated movement makes for an efficient, accessible class. In the Sun Salutations framework, you can repeat some of the postures within it to maximize foundations.

- Repeat the half-Sun Salutations a few times
- Repeat moving from Downward-facing Dog to Plank pose (in a class with moderate to higher levels of mobility, assuming students are okay on their wrists)
- Repeat the Cobra pose (*Bhujangasana*) multiple times
- On the belly, lift into and out of Locust pose (*Salabhasana*) with the inhalations and come to the ground on the exhalations
- Add back or shoulder strengthening by lying on the belly (prone position) with props or with repeated arm movements

Replace Plank pose (*Phalakasana*). Many people can step back to Downward-facing Dog, but the push-up position is too challenging.

Take out the Plank pose and prone positions altogether, and instead try the following substitutions.

- Step back to Downward-facing Dog, and then come to hands and knees for Tabletop pose activities
- Instead of Cobra pose, do "bird dogs" (lift a leg and the opposite arm, lower, repeat with alternate leg and arm, continue the pattern), or any number of core activities you can do from hands and knees
- Your pregnant students will be so grateful not to be on their bellies or doing yet another Cat/Cow pose (*Marjaryasana/Bitilasana*)!

If the forward folding is aggravating for blood pressure or balance, explore movement standing up.

- Try moving into and out of Chair pose (*Utkatasana*) at varying angles; you can hold a block between the legs as well
- Explore flexion and extension of the spine organically
- Replace Sun Salutations altogether by adding warming work into each body position, alternating with calm activities (you won't miss them!)

Here's an example of a Sun Salutation alternative for you. This would work particularly well if you have a class that can get up and down easily, have some familiarity with sun salutations, but you want to increase the accessibility and efficiency.

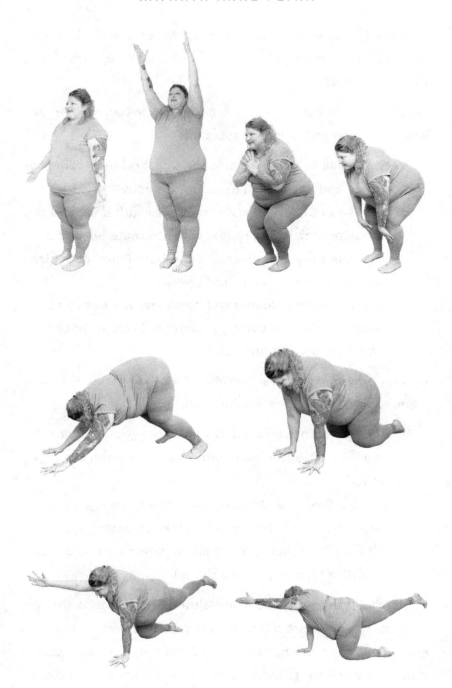

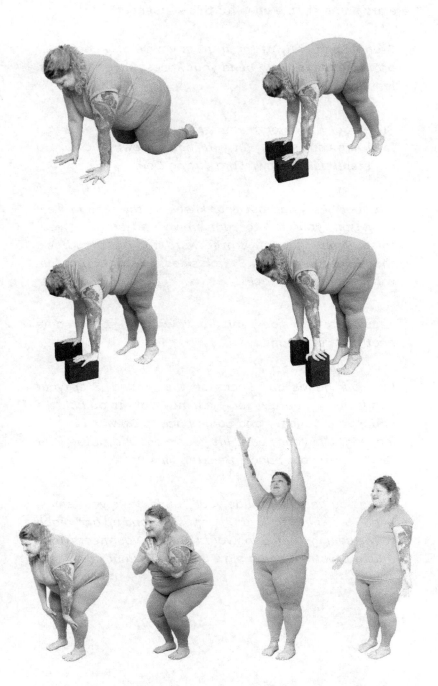

Here are some simple cues for this sequence:

Stand confidently at the front of your mat. Reach your arms overhead...now bend your knees, hands to heart, land in Chair pose.

Slide your hands onto your shins, look forward as you lengthen your spine. Put your hands down and take a big step back to Downward-facing Dog.

Lift your heels and put your knees on the ground. Feel long from your tail to your crown and stabilize your torso. Reach your left arm forward and right leg back, then float them down. Switch sides, with right arm forward and left leg back.

Keep switching sides, mindfully, while we build some heat and core stability.

Put your hands and knees on the ground. Step your hands apart a little wider – you may want to add blocks under your hands – and come back to Downward-facing Dog. Lift your heels, lift your hips, and tiptoe your feet toward your hands. Hips up, hips up!

When you get there, slide your hands on to your shins, bend your knees toward Chair pose. Stand up and reach to the ceiling, then bring your hands to your heart. Take a long breath in and a slow breath out your nose.

Journaling Activity

Plan a Sun Salutation that subtracts Plank pose and Upward-facing Dog and replaces them with something else that is warming and strengthening and involves lying on the belly.

Plan another Sun Salutation (again, without Plank and Upward-facing Dog) that would be appropriate for yogis who cannot lie on their bellies.

PART FIVE

Teaching Yoga

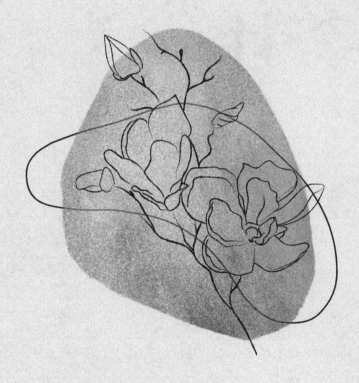

TEACHING YOGA AND PRACTICING yoga are two different skill sets. During your teacher training, you may remember your first invitation to cue a yoga posture, and the surprise you experienced trying to describe Downward Facing Dog. It is surprising how challenging it can be to describe in words something you have done in your body thousands of times.

Unlike the physical aspect of practice however, our teaching only develops scope with time. Dramatic or high-mobility yoga postures will fall away from our practice long before we might retire from teaching. The progression of teachers is much like our progression as students—we begin with the body, but it becomes so much more about the mind and spirit as we go on.

This section includes methods and concepts like earlier sections, but if you are already teaching yoga, introducing new concepts may feel particularly foreign to your current methods. My suggestion is that you pick a few new ideas and work with them—another commitment to the testing, observing, and re-testing approach to yoga.

Sequencing

IN THE UPCOMING "CUEING" section of the book, I compare the components of cueing a class to a recipe. Cueing and sequencing interweave to create the practice atmosphere. If we extend the recipe metaphor, the class sequences are the ingredients and the outcome of your recipe. Some elements share little in common, but in combination, they create an excellent result.

Most of the advice in this section centers on the movement content of your classes, but that is not the only lens we bring to our *yoga-asana*. We begin by considering the *qualities* different components generate, and turn to Ayurveda again for its wisdom.

The Qualities of Yoga-Asana

One of my friend and teacher Mona's books is *Āyurvedic Yoga: 3 Approaches to Teaching Āyurvedic Yoga*, which gives yogis an excellent foundation in teaching yoga from an Ayurvedic perspective—one that harmonizes practice and the needs of the season.

As mentioned at the beginning of this book, Ayurveda dictates that nature is comprised of five elements (ether, air, fire, water, and earth) and each of these elements has its own particular qualities (*guna*) to describe how it functions. Each season has two elements that govern it, and so we are more affected by those elements and experience their *gunas* more powerfully, especially if we have a lot of those particular elements in our own composition (*prakriti*).

For example, springtime is governed by water and earth, which have the qualities of heaviness, stickiness (earth + water = mud!), and coolness. That means that physically and psychologically we will struggle with heaviness (slow to get going, feelings of lethargy or depression), stickiness (slow digestion, inability to let go of certain thoughts or beliefs), and coolness (damp, clammy body).

Mona writes, "We can either figure out how to teach a technique to increase one quality or the other, or figure out which techniques fit on which side of the continuum." Qualities exist on a continuum, because they are mostly paired into opposites. The qualities of Ayurveda are:

heavy (*guru*) / light (*laghu*)
slow or dull (*manda*) / sharp or penetrating (*tiksna*)
cold (*hima* or *sita*) / hot (*usna*)
oily or unctuous (*snigdha* or *sneha*) / dry (*ruksa*)
smooth (*slaksna*) / rough (*khara*)
soft (*mrdu*) / hard (*kathina*)

stable (*sthira*) / mobile or unstable (*cala*)

gross or big or obvious (*sthula*) / subtle (*suksma*)

cloudy or slimy or sticky (*picchila*) / clear (*visada*)

If the season is characterized by coolness, we can do a practice that removes the root cause of coolness, or a practice that warms us up if the cause cannot be removed (though we may wish away winter, it will continue to come back!).

I highly suggest reading Mona's books for more specific information on how to teach Ayurvedic yoga, but you can begin here by thinking about the qualities promoted by each activity/posture in your sequences, and the overall effect of your sequence. Here are a couple of examples.

Seated Forward Folds

Seated forward folds could cultivate grounding (heaviness and stability), so it would be unusual to place a lengthily held seated forward fold in the middle of your active class sequence. In its stillness our heart rates would decrease, which would cool us off.

That would be too much heaviness and coolness for a portion of class that needs movement and heat.

However, if you teach it in a way that is assertive and goal-oriented—think cueing "nose to toes"—you would promote hard-headedness (*kathina*) and heat through the striving.

How you teach something is as important as *what* you teach, so marry your intentions and content together.

Kapalabhati Pranayama

As outlined in the "Pranayama" section later in the book, this *pranayama* is invigorating—it makes our energy move (*cala*)—and heating (*usna*). If we teach it in a really hot room at the end of class when yogis are dry from perspiration (*ruksa*), it may overly dry us up, or heat us up to the point of developing fiery minds!

Taught after a warm-up, but before the standing portion of a sequence, the mobilizing energy and sharpness (*tiksna*) of this *pranayama* could help us cut through the brain fog and physical lethargy we may bring to class, and act as excellent preparation for paying attention during our standing sequence.

Journaling Activity

Write down five of your favorite yoga activities—they could be postures or exercises. Now, look at the list of Ayurveda's qualities (*gunas*). What qualities might these activities increase or decrease? Where would they best be placed in a sequence?

These are unusual sequencing choices. Write down what qualities these activities promote, and consider when you might make this sequencing choice.

1. A 5-minute *Savasana* just after the middle of class
2. Beginning class with a supported backbend
3. Beginning class with a standing sequence
4. Doing repetitions of X number for several activities

Sequencing Classes

When we sequence classes, we are considering the movement capabilities of the bodies in the room, the desired effects of each posture and their cumulative effect as a sequence, postures that require warm-up/mental preparation, class duration, and class structure, all while aiming to leave sufficient time to wind down and integrate with *Savasana* or another integrative pose.

Whether you are sequencing a complicated journey between and toward advanced postures or offering a very accessible class, these principles will help you guide your students with confidence and compassion. Yoga classes do not have to sacrifice strengthening and mobilizing for accessibility, and I hope that this material has helped you see how that is possible.

Here are some principles for keeping your classes accessible while still increasing their efficiency.

Follow the class structure arc of ground → standing/crouching → ground, because coming up and down between postures with different foundations is tricky.

Reducing the number of times you come up to stand is essential, so if you follow this class structure arc, you can maximize the standing sequence. How many times you come up to stand depends on the mobility of the people in the room. You have to think beyond linking postures with half a breath cycle (like Vinyasa-style classes) when you are aiming to be inclusive.

Of course, you can start your classes from seated or standing position. Still, in my experience, it is easier to structure an accessible class sequence around a gradual rise up and gradual return to the floor in body position than when I start elsewhere. I also prefer not to do heating core work right before *Savasana*, which sometimes happens when yoga teachers only teach reclined postures as class ends.

Journaling Activity

What is a four-posture/activity sequence that you like to open a practice with? Why do you like it— is it grounding energetically, stretching across your chest or hips, or warming up?

What is a four-posture/activity sequence that you like to incorporate in the middle of practice? What do you like about it?

What is a two- or three-posture/activity sequence that you like to use to wind down practice? What do these wind-down activities offer you?

Reduce transitions and add movement within postures.

Remember, even simple movements require a multi-segmental (multi-joint) response of both mobility (functional range) and stability (prevention of movement). Some transitions between postures involve quite complicated movements. When we reduce transitions *between* poses and add movement *within* positions, we increase accessibility.

Journaling Activity

What are three postures you know that you like adding movement to? Are there any other movements you could do with each of them?

Alternate between movement and stillness.

As efficient as adding movement within postures can be, we also want to witness the harmonious flow of *prana* and internalize our practice, rather than merely trying to wring every moment for utility. Make sure there are elements of stillness-in-posture throughout.

Increase eccentric/concentric contraction in standing and seated postures to strengthen the upper body with less wrist compression.

When we think of shoulder/core strengthening in yoga, we may go too quickly to Vinyasa flows or Plank poses *(Phalakasana)*. Instead, you can integrate shoulder strength with props and encourage movement and varied contractions *beyond* isometric contractions. Some people are even incorporating resistance bands and weights into their yoga classes.

Reduce opportunities for wrist compression.

Earlier in the book, we listed setup tricks for reducing wrist compression. Here are sequencing tricks.

- Replace the Plank *(Phalakasana)*/Upward-facing Dog *(Urdhva Mukha Svanasana)* of Sun Salutations with hands-and-knees positions, which still involve a flexed wrist, but with less body weight placed on the joint
- Punctuate activities in hands/knees positions with either forearms down (forearm Plank or Dolphin [*Ardha Pincha Mayurasana*]) or lying prone on the belly
- Test your students' wrist-readiness by having them bring their forearms and palms together, stretch their fingers back, and if they can't make a "T" shape, they will need the yoga wedge approach and should reduce/eliminate Plank poses (you should try this too, and hold it for a few moments!)

Swap complicated *yoga-asana* for exercises/activities that break down the components.

There are lots of gorgeous yoga postures out there, and while some people in your class may be able to do them, many will not. For example, Revolved Triangle *(Parivrtta Trikonasana)* pose requires a lot of flexibility and mobility, including a knee extension with complex hip rotation, spinal extension, etc. To incorporate a pose like this (or elements of it), build up to it with movements that promote twisting well, extending legs well, etc., and then teach a levelled version of the more complex posture. You can always use props to increase stability and form.

Increase the amount of time spent on your back.

There are a lot of great exercises that can be done while on the back. Since the torso contains a lot of stabilizing muscles, we want to strengthen them without aggravating the joints of the hands/feet. Being on the back reduces that risk! This is a great way to work on strengthening if you have any concerns about your students' spinal health.

Increase the amount of time spent on hands and knees and seated.

Yes, I did say to watch out for wrist compression, but on the hands and knees is a great position to work from because it provides firm boundaries that will help us direct the force of contraction in the ways we want to. There are many activities you can do in a seated position too, and you have the added benefit of getting to look at your students and do a bit of well-placed demonstrating to build up the community vibe. For students who cannot spend time on hands and knees, experiment with variations in seated – they work well!

Learn how to sequence around fatiguing one part of the body.

If you watch your students through the practice, you will learn reasonable lengths of time to work people in specific positions. In my "Accessible Yoga Teacher Training" course for existing yoga teachers, the participants are often shocked to find out that my classes are peppy, not demoralizing. They often find the classes quite challenging, which surprises them because, to many people, "accessible" implies "easy."

To experience a "peppy, not demoralizing" class, go to www.kathrynanneflynn.com

Overlooked Activities

When I review practice teaches during teacher training, I can often tell the yoga school and style a student usually practices with, since we typically draw on our own experiences to sequence our first classes. Regardless of where the student has practiced though, I consistently notice that there are a few things students often exclude when trying to deliver a well-rounded class.

A lot of these exclusions happen, I believe, because of the popularity of yoga. Since so many yoga students have no intention of honing a yoga and movement practice beyond weekly yoga, many do not have the prerequisite mobility to perform some beneficial yoga activities. When students cannot do these activities, teachers may just eliminate them without replacing the missing material with activities that are similar and accessible.

This list is to help you contemplate what you might be missing while you are trying to teach an accessible yoga class.

Hands and Wrists, Feet, and Ankles

Warming up the smaller muscles of the body, especially when they are so important for interacting with the world, is important for safe movement.

It can be as simple as reaching hands and feet to the ceiling and rolling the wrists and ankles for a while, switching directions to maintain balance. Your toolkit of these types of activities will likely never be as unique as some of your other activities, but they do not need to be interesting, just effective.

Active Stretching Backbends

Some of the more active stretching backbends, like Camel *(Ustrasana)*, Wheel *(Chakrasana)*, and Bow pose *(Dhanurasana)*, are not accessible. Many people cannot reach the ground behind them, even in lower variations of Camel, so here are a few active stretching activities that give us an active stretch across the front of the chest and shoulders without excluding some students.

Remember, even seated backbends should be accompanied with gentle reminders for full and slow breath. Postures are containers for watching the movement of breath.

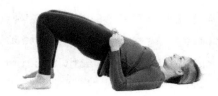

Robot Arm Bridge

This Bridge pose *(Setu Bandha Sarvangasana)* uses "robot arms" – elbows bent at 90 degrees with closed fists. Hands can stay open, but closed fists help with the downward engagement of your upper arms. The "typical" Bridge pose requires extended elbows and sometimes interlaced fingers. Achieving that bind can limit the external rotation in your shoulders. The bent elbows prevent internal rotation and allow for broadening across your chest muscles.

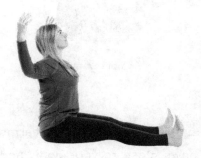

Cactus Arm Backbend

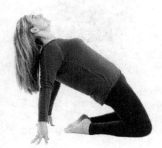

Camel Variation

Cactus Arm Backbend

Sit with your legs loosely extended. "Cactus" your arms at shoulder height. Stretch your elbows back as you lift your chest and lift your chin, then hold for a few breaths. In the Awesome-a section, this is one part of a movement. Many movement activities have elements that can be held as a pose.

Camel Variation

Kneeling with knees wide, place your hands on the ground behind you or on blocks. I enjoy incorporating both flat palms and tented fingers for diversity. As you lift your hips, experiment with squeezing your bum, lengthening your rib cage, lengthening from your knees to your waist, and broadening across your chest. Your head can stay forward, or go back.

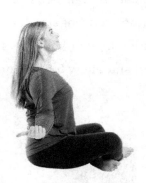 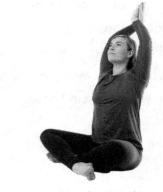

Seated Backbend with Funky Thumbs   Temple Stretch

Seated Backbend with Funky Thumbs

Sit cross-legged and do two thumbs up. With your forearms out by your sides, keep your elbows close to your body, and squeeze your upper arms back as you round your chest. Rotate your thumbs and feel like they're reaching to the space behind you.

Temple Stretch

Sitting cross legged, lift your arms overhead and cross at the wrists to place your palms against each other. Pressing your palms into each other, bend your elbows. You can lift your heartspace and feel your sides lengthen.

Bent-Elbow Shoulder Extension

You will often see twists performed like the picture below— one arm bent to hold a leg, and the other arm straightened up behind you.

Many people perform the classical yoga twist Half Lord of the Fishes (*Ardha Matsyendrasana*) with a straight arm. As

I'm demonstrating here, students sometimes lean into their straight arm and flat palm, making half the posture quite relaxed and unintentional.

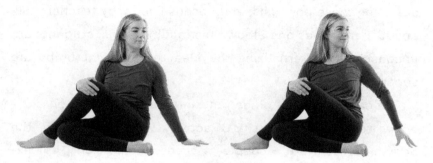

Half Lord of the Fishes (*Ardha Matsy-endrasana*) with a straight arm

Half Lord of the Fishes (*Ardha Matsy-endrasana*) with a bent elbow

However, exploring this pose with a bent elbow is also useful, because it promotes alignment of the spine and more intentional embodiment of the back and arm muscles.

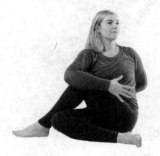

Another interesting variation is to sandwich yourself in two bent arms, squeezing your legs and torso between them.

As yoga in the West has become more inclusive, fewer people are moving toward practicing the binds of classical *yoga-asana*—the arms linked around a leg to join hands.

It's a very different shoulder position that first requires a bent elbow and then takes the arm into a strong internal rotation and shoulder extension position. Because fewer people are doing these positions, and because so many teachers talk about "bent knees and elbows" as modifications, students are unconsciously internalizing the idea that straight limbs are superior.

We can work "half binds" and integrate this position elsewhere to promote diversity of activity, which is good for the bodymind. Here are a couple of accessible versions, but experiment on your own to see where they make sense.

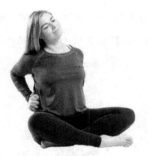

Bound Neck Stretch

Settle into your preferred sitting position. Reach your left arm behind your back and hold your hand, wrist, or forearm with your right hand. Tip your head toward your right shoulder, and feel like you're breathing into the left side of your neck. Linger for several breaths before releasing, doing some gentle movement, and moving on to the other side.

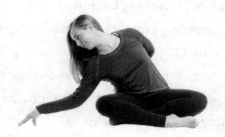

Sit cross-legged and reach your left arm behind your back. You can hold on to your shirt, press your hand into your back, or hold on to your pants. Put the fingertips of your right hand on the floor out to your right side and walk them up. Side bend toward your right hand, keeping your left arm behind you. You can always reach your left arm overhead for a couple of breaths too, before doing the other side.

Core Work Emphasizing Suppleness and Strength

The core work of more classical Hatha yoga requires that you be able to move your abdominal muscles skillfully, which includes relaxing and controlling them. If you are interested in treading the classical yoga path to optimally functional abdominal muscles, it begins with *Dirgha Pranayama* (the long breath), continues with *Kapalabhati* (shining skull breath), moves on to *Agni Sara* (fire essence), and then *Nauli* (abdominal churning).

Since these activities require a high level of commitment, they are not taught in typical yoga classes. Yoga teachers have borrowed from other exercise fields to include abdominal and core strengthening exercises, but they tend to emphasize attaining flatness and strength in the region.

Including active stretching backbends will help, as will taking the time to properly practice and teach *Dirgha Pranayama*. You can also do this Bridge pose (*Setu Bandha Sarvangasana*) rolling activity with an emphasis on movement in the abdomen. You may want to demonstrate this one before class begins and explain the goals of the pose.

Caution, it is not for all students: As the position requires the breath to be held after exhalation, offer students for whom breath retention is not appropriate to continue with Flowing Bridge pose, or offer them a pranayama practice, such as supine or seated *Dirgha Pranayama* with their hands on their abdomen. Students who are pregnant, who suffer from anxiety and/or unstable emotions, who have high blood pressure, have undergone recent surgery, and those who have eye conditions should not practice *Uddiyana Bandha*.

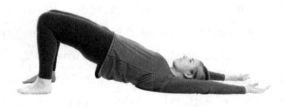

Bridge pose with arms overhead.

Begin with a supine warm-up and then some Flowing Bridge, rolling up and down the spine with flowing arms. Pause in Overhead Bridge pose with arms up, and exhale dramatically with semi-pursed lips, trying to make a wind gust noise.

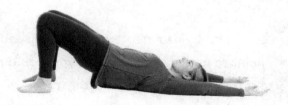

Bridge pose with arms overhead and belly drawn
up and under.

Relaxing the abdomen as much as possible, hold the exhalation out and "fly" the diaphragm and belly tissues under the rib cage (Uddiyana Bandha).

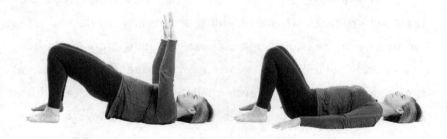

Rolling down with diaphragm drawn up under rib cage.

Slowly roll to the ground as you hold the exhalation, with a special emphasis on moving sequentially down the spine, and calmly breathe in once arrived. You can experiment with holding the exhalation here and then calmly breathing in when you feel it is time. If you are gasping for air, you are holding for too long.

Repeat a few times before relaxing on the ground, observing the breath.

Mini Sequences

If you were to attend a seasoned teacher's classes frequently and made a point to notice their content, you would pick up on their repertoire of mini-sequences. Often they are postures/ activities that build upon each other, complement each other, or maximize the body position to reduce tricky transitions between poses.

Now, if you are teaching a roomful of people who can get up and down off the ground with ease, that in itself has become a movement activity. You can see videos and suggestions for such exercises all over the internet! However, if you are teaching students with a diversity of mobility levels and trying to offer accessible yoga classes, reducing transitions between body positions is a necessary component. The activities themselves can still be plenty challenging for even the skillful movers in the room. Nevertheless, students with severe arthritis, a replaced knee, high blood pressure, etc., will be grateful to not be left behind by rapid transitions between positions. The following suggestions might inspire you to add such mini-sequences to your own classes.

1. Mini-sequences that develop similar movements/ engagements/alignment
   * Warrior II (*Virabhadrasana II*) → Extended Side Angle (*Utthita Parsvakonasana*) → Half Moon (*Ardha Chandrasana*)

- Plank (*Phalakasana*) → Forearm Plank (*Phalakasana variation*) → Forearm Side Plank (*Vasisthasana variation*)
- Mountain *(Tadasana)* → Chair (*Utkatasana*)→ Revolved Chair (*Parivrtta Utkatasana*)

2. "High-efficiency" sequences that get complementary activities done from one place
   - Seated twist → Seated side bend → Forward fold (over crossed legs)
   - Warrior I (*Virabhadrasana* I) → Shoulder work with block → Humble Warrior variation (*Baddha Virabhadrasana*)
   - Hip mobility exercise → Stag pose → Pigeon variation (*Kapotasana variation*)

3. Sequences that lead into and out of a particular posture
   - Dolphin *(Ardha Pincha Mayurasana)* → Headstand *(Sirsasana)* → Thread the Needle *(Parsva Balasana)* → Shoulder Release
   - Flowing Bridge *(Setu Bandha Sarvangasana)* → Bridge with leg lifts → Hamstring stretch → Reclined twist

Do Yoga Postures Need to Be Countered?

In my yoga teacher training program we teach participants to sequence their yoga classes through discussion, group work, and individual planning. They use the sequencing guidelines you will find in this book.

One of the most common clarifications I need to make in every training course is that of including counter yoga postures. Yoga postures do not need to be "countered"—that is, a posture that takes the body into one range of movement does not need to pair with another particular posture.

This has not always been the case, as yoga sequencing centered on this concept for a long time. To show how my understanding has evolved, I left the outdated ideas in my program manual and added notes showing the evolution of thought. It is helpful to acknowledge our own journey of refinement.

Warm-up and preparation are more important than counter postures. If you are going to do a significantly challenging yoga posture, like Wheel pose (*Chakrasana*), you have to warm everyone up with a sequence that includes shoulder flexion, more moderate backbends, wrist preparation, and hip extension.

After Wheel pose, there is no need to do a deep forward fold or Plough pose *(Halasana)*. As we have explored, the feelings of stretch are quite fleeting; they will dissipate as you calm down and remove the loads on specific tissues (i.e., when the posture is over).

You may have heard yoga teachers talk about "the burning sensation" in muscles, which is lactic acid buildup that accompanies intense activity. Your muscles' first fuel is oxygen (aerobic), but when the oxygen supply runs low during physical activity, they rely on pyruvate, which has been converted from the bloodstream's glucose for energy (anaerobic). When the body has less oxygen than it needs to perform aerobically, lactic acid accumulates as a by-product of the anaerobic process, allowing for glucose conversion for another 1–3 minutes (causing the burning sensation).

If you stop doing that activity, the feelings will dissipate. The burning sensation goes away without further intervention.

Some postures may feel pleasant following another, but we may need to invite students to resist the reactive clutching or immediate twisting after a yoga posture. The reactivity can exacerbate feelings of "there is a problem that needs to be relieved," rather than learning to ride the waves of non-harmful feelings of the body. We need to feel the effects of the work we've done!

When I teach Bridge pose *(Setu Bandha Sarvangasana)*, I invite students to lay on the ground, rest their hands on the body, and feel themselves breathe slowly, "allowing the posture to integrate."

As yoga students, we are learning to discern between feelings that are harmful to us, and feelings that are passing and non-harmful. Letting students know that counter postures are not required can open the door to learning to self-calm and regulate with calm breathing and reflection.

Dare to Be Simple

A couple of years ago, a graduate from my foundational yoga program attended class with me for the first time in a while. Upon exit, he said, "Thank you for the reminder that spaciousness is not the opposite of efficient."

What a change from my early days, when I thought complexity and borderline-alienating Vinyasa formed the path to success! Now I teach to the person in the room with the lowest level of mobility, even if everyone else could execute gymnastics. I teach progressive levels and choose a specific style to avoid glorifying extreme flexibility, which, as we have learned, will not always result in being pain-free. These approaches offer an experience that acknowledges the unique individuals in the room while still honoring a community practice.

Since repetition helps build heat, and we promote accessibility with repetitive, simple activities, we have to share the benefits of repetition and simplicity. We can remind students that consistency over time trumps intensity. We can tell them that the brain pays less attention to what it *thinks* it knows, and the repetition of movements is an invitation to mindfulness practice.

Movement practice is healthy for our tissues, the flow of our energy, and our mental outlook; it reveals habitual thought patterns that show up when we are bored or overwhelmed. This is part of why people call yoga a moving meditation—not because our upstairs is blank and empty, but because what shows up in our inner awareness reveals a lot about our habituated thoughts.

Accessible yoga sequencing that includes repetitive movements and functional movement exercises can often feel less "fancy" than the Vinyasa sequencing that led to yoga's popularity explosion. Performing fancy postures, sequences, and even mobility exercises like pistol squats can come from a place of aesthetic achievement. Healthy movement exploration can feel beautiful, but it can also feel boring, like oatmeal (good for us, but not exactly great Instagram content). When we can learn to accept feelings of boredom and frustration as an element of responsible practice, we can cultivate self-compassion and experience greater ease, on and off the yoga mat.

In the same way that you eat some meals week to week that are "old reliables," but still try new things as well, it is the diversity that matters.

I have supervised many, many practice teaches in yoga teacher training, so let me reassure you that "simplicity, but executed well" trumps "fancy, but executed poorly." Some people practice the same yoga postures for their entire yoga career! Dare to be simple.

Overall Class Structure

We've learned that we have to remember to include some overlooked activities, and that we can sequence multiple segments of class by thinking of mini-sequences within larger sequences. Zooming out even further, we now look at overall class structure.

Class structure is a lot like a narrative arc: opening, establishing the facts, rising action, climax, denouement, and conclusion.

Remember that you may alternate between standing and floor postures as they may make sense, but maximize the amount of time you have in each body position!

For typical class lengths, breakdowns could look like the suggestions below.

Savasana Alert: Getting people into and out of *Savasana* takes longer than you may suspect, especially in a room-temperature setting where students might have socks/sweaters/props. In hot yoga classes, people tend to just flop to the mat, but at room temperature, they lovingly take the time to get cozy. A 15-minute *Savasana* only achieves 8–10 minutes of everyone in *Savasana* at the same time, because getting students back up to a seated position in a calm, kind fashion takes a few minutes.

Class: 60 minutes

A 60-minute class offers the opportunity for a well-rounded practice without extras (peak postures, workshop-approach within class, etc.). Design your classes with a focus on diverse programming that produces a holistic effect on the bodymind. Themes and peak postures can be introduced as you feel more confident guiding students into them with ease and minimal set up.

- 20 minutes of opening/invitation to awareness, floor work, and preparatory activities (wrist strengthening, opening stretches, core work, etc.)

- 20 minutes of standing and crouching postures (Sun Salutation variations, standing sequence poses like Warrior(s) or Goddess, mobility exercises, and standing balance postures)
- 10 minutes of floor work (*pranayama*, seated stretching)
- 10 minutes of final restorative pose and *Savasana*

Class: 75 minutes

Seventy-five minutes is a common length for a class, as it provides time for a well-rounded practice, a little bit of extra attention to one activity, and a good *Savasana*.

- 20 minutes of opening breathwork, cultivating awareness, floor work and preparatory activities
- 35 minutes of standing and crouching postures
- 10 minutes of *pranayama* or specific *asana* focus (workshop) or mobility exercise
- 10–15 minutes of floor work
- 10–15 minutes of final cool down poses and *Savasana* or integration

Class: 90 minutes

This class length is a great amount of time; providing space for diverse programming without feeling rushed.

- 30 minutes of opening, breathwork, cultivating awareness, floor work, and details
- 10 minutes of a gradual build into standing (crouching postures)

- 25–30 minutes of standing, crouching postures, peak postures and even wall work (using the wall for standing stretches or supported hip stretches from the back)
- 10–15 minutes of floor work
- 15–20 minutes of *Savasana*

Fluffing Your Cotton Ball

Yes, you read that section title correctly! This sequencing recommendation would best be understood if you have a cotton ball in your hands, so please go retrieve one and then be patient (if you don't have one, I'm sure you can imagine one).

Earlier in the book, I mention that if we were going to have a metaphor for the way biological tissues function, we would use silly putty. However, cotton balls are cheaper, more easily found in your home, and my toddler is less interested in them (i.e., my silly putty keeps going missing). *Hang on to your cotton ball for a moment.*

If we are walking bundles of cells, and those cells are spherical, then perhaps we can look to a spherical item as a better metaphor for movement self-care than the angles, towers, and lines of mechanics.

If you were to teach a class that just emphasized the extension of the knee and stretching (hamstring stretching), you would only be fluffing one part of the ball. *Go ahead and only fluff up one part of the ball.*

When your movement practice is predominantly one kind of activity—only weight-lifting, only cardio, only stretching, only bouncing (assuming someone is doing that)—you are only fluffing one part of the ball.

If you wanted to fluff the whole ball...how would you go about that? *Try it and report back.*

My guess is that you steadily, mindfully, and somewhat playfully, moved your way around the cotton ball and evenly fluffed each bit of it. This is how we approach sequencing in my classes and trainings—we seek to evenly fluff your ball. A diversity of movement content, exploration, and a spirit of playfulness keeps you and your metaphorical ball fluffy. Keep your fluffed cotton ball to inspire your programming.

Class Content Checklist

A well-rounded class seeks to do a lot in a relatively short amount of time—it seeks to fluff your ball with high efficiency. This can be intimidating for a new teacher, but just remember that any amount of movement, stillness, and conscious breathing is good. You will get better at delivering a class in the same way you got better at knowing how to do a class.

When you are looking at the sequences that you've developed, consider the little transitions in between things, but overall, look for diversity in experience and for movement. A well-rounded class combines a balance of activities that deliver these elements.

Sequencing Activity: Take a look at your class plans and check off the element each activity satisfies—it may be more than one. This will reveal to you if your practice has no backbending, too much forward folding, is overall too peppy, etc.

Atmosphere

Supportive and contemplative
Activity details, directions and education
Silence

Energy

Invigorating
Smoothing/fluidity
Down-regulating (calming)

Activity

Stillness
Still stretching
Active stretching
Mobility exercises
Strengthening
Exploratory/Workshop style
Endurance/reflective
Pranayama/Breath focus
Integration/Meditation

Body Positioning

Prone front
Supine back
Crouching
Standing
Balancing

Directions of the Spine, Shoulders, and Hips

Backbends
Side bends
Forward folds
Twists
Elongation
Overhead arms (shoulder flexion)
Arms back and behind (shoulder extension)
Knees closer to chest (hip flexion)
Knees away from waist (hip extension)
Legs apart, legs together
One side at a time (unilateral)
Both sides at a time (bilateral)

...plus all the variations on these, like elbows bent, extended, arms in front, behind, etc.

From a movement perspective, you want a diversity of joint articulations with varying forces and loads moved throughout the body.

Peak Postures

A popular sequencing technique in Vinyasa classes is "peak posture" sequencing, where the sequence is designed to prepare students for a posture that requires significant mental effort, flexibility, and strength.

These days I devote most of my "time heavy" class activities to supported backbends, but if you are interested in teaching peak postures and tricky classes, consider these tips to set your students up for success.

1. Consider the warm-ups required for the complex joints your students will be using, and sequence postures around their preparation.
   a. Example: Working toward Bird of Paradise (*Svarga Dvijasana*), you would need to start with:
      i. Hamstring extension
      ii. Hip flexion and external rotation
      iii. General warmth through hips/core
      iv. Shoulder extension with elbow flexion (bind position)
2. Warm folks up sufficiently without alienating students who are newer or who have a lower mobility level *and* leave enough gas in the tank for everyone to try the posture
3. Understand how to offer a leveled experience of the posture so everyone has a meaningful option

4. Be familiar with the pose's challenges and ways of working with them (i.e., consider challenges beyond your
own—talk to people!)

Give time for calm exploration. Innovation needs to make
sense and requires time for students to get into/out of it, so
it will not happen at the pace of a flow sequence. Exploration and execution can take more time than you'd anticipate—
schedule in minutes, not moments.

Make Tricky Sequences More Accessible

Carving out time for yogis to try a tricky balance is easier to
make inclusive than a continuous flowing class. There are
some yoga sequences and postures that are achievable for
more people if you simply slow them down, but some transitions are just too quick to be accessible and safe. However, if
you teach in a class with students who have higher mobility
levels and want to *improve* the accessibility of your classes,
you may be surprised at what folks are capable of if you prepare them with information and suitable options.

For example, the below sequence is extremely difficult and
should not be offered in a class labeled as accessible, but
taken slowly, and with modifications offered, it is more accessible than you may think.

This sequence is built around these postures and transitions:

* Warrior I *(Virabhadrasana I)*
* Supported Side Plank or Side Plank *(Vasisthasana)*

- Forearm Side Plank (*Vasisthasana variation*)
- Finishing in Forearm Plank (*Phalakasana variation*)

It alternates "sides"—Warrior I with left foot forward, Side Plank with right hand down, Forearm Side Plank with left forearm down, and then Forearm Plank.

To begin, warm up with this variation of Sun Salutations:

- Half Sun Salutation (*Ardha Surya Namaskar*)
- Warrior I *(Virabhdrasana I)*
- Downward-facing Dog *(Adho Mukha Svanasana)*
- Plank (with knees down) *(Phalakasana)*
- Forearm Plank (with knees down) *(Phalakasana variation)*
- Sphinx pose *(Salamaba Bhujangasana)*

Forearm Plank pose is more accessible than you'd think—it develops trunk stability, being close to the ground makes for easy/inconspicuous rest breaks, and beyond requiring toe extension, it does not tax small muscles or joints. Some people may need a towel placed on the mat so their elbows are comfortable, but otherwise, many people can at least do a knees-down variation.

Offering Sphinx pose after the first Forearm Plank also cultivates permission for putting one's body on the ground, rather than powering through.

When you teach this variation on the Sun Salutation, you remind your class that you are going to start mixing in other postures like Side Plank, and they can keep repeating the Forearm Plank/Sphinx pose sequence. This is also a good sequence to demonstrate before class starts to reassure people that there are multiple options.

Yogis can then do the first sequence, or:

- Warrior I to Plank to Forearm Plank (with knees down)
  - Teach people how to engage their musculature in knees-down Forearm Plank by asking them to lengthen their lower back by zipping into high-waisted jeans while simultaneously trying (and not succeeding) to pull their knees and elbows toward each other

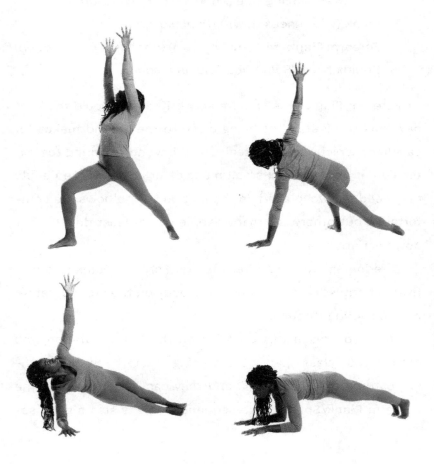

- Repeat, then add in Side Plank with one foot support option (Warrior I to Side Plank with foot support to Forearm Plank)
- Repeat, then add in Forearm Side Plank after Side Plank, and then head into Forearm Plank (Warrior I to Side Plank to Forearm Plank on the opposite arm to Forearm Plank)

By the time you go through the sequence with all the options, people will move more fluidly into the proper shapes because, like a dance routine, they have learned the steps. You will also have your entire standing sequence completed! One version of the sequence might look this: Warrior I, Supported Side Plank, Forearm Side Plank, Forearm Plank.

One caveat: *This sequence doesn't work for lower- to average-mobility populations.* There's just too much up/down movement. Reserve this sequence for a setting where you are teaching a class with a higher level of mobility, but also with a diversity of students in attendance.

Getting up and getting down on the mat is challenging for a lot of people, and it is one of the primary reasons that a sequence might be inaccessible. It takes strength and balance through the whole movement. Literally getting up and down can be a good mobility practice, but in a *yoga-asana* setting, you want to reduce these instances for an accessible yoga class.

Cueing

TEACHING YOGA IS A complicated public speaking job. While delivering a list of instructions with clarity, empowerment, and inspiration, you are simultaneously assessing the visual feedback of bodies moving through the interpretation of those instructions.

Sometimes yoga teachers disproportionately focus on the empowerment element. This could be a result of their own transformative experiences with yoga. They prioritize learning the inspirational speech elements of teaching a class, such as an opening talk about the theme, encouragement to keep going, or creatively describing movement in ways that are visually evocative, like "rooting down through the legs and blossoming up through the arms."

When you focus too many cues on generating "magic moments" instead of teaching movement with clarity, your outcome might be confusion.

Inspiration is absolutely a part of teaching a good yoga class, but clearly and effectively moving people around a yoga mat through exercises, stretches, and breathwork is the requisite framework for inspiration. You cannot gift wrap a box until the box is built—yoga classes need to deliver the minimum promise of a clear, mindful, movement and breath experience before you have a foundation for inspiration.

Teaching Like a Cooking Show

We can look to the kitchen to inspire our framework. Yoga classes can be cued the way a recipe provides instructions— combining elements and finessing techniques in an order that results in reasonable success. Translating words into movement is tricky, so when we deliver our cues like a recipe— ordered explicitly for a specific result—we are more likely to achieve clarity.

From the yoga teacher's perspective, a well-cued yoga class can be more mundane than magic, because delivering the instructions is different than experiencing them. To come back to our box metaphor, you know how tricky it can be to get the details right for a beautifully wrapped package, but the opener of the present appreciates the method without analyzing it. Your students do not notice the repetition of simple movement cues, but they do notice how confused they feel when cues are unclear. Skillful methods are often invisible.

The cues that inspire us, the uplifting words that speak right to our spirit—that artistry cannot be appreciated unless the infrastructure of a clear, steady practice is in place.

Students tell me that they appreciate the clarity and consistency with which I teach my classes, which should permit you to *be repetitive*. While I have indeed evolved my cues over the years (and as I've encountered communities with different needs), I am incredibly repetitive. When you teach, you may feel extra repetitive because you say the same instructions frequently, but those words facilitate movement and experiences that elude words.

There is beauty in simplicity. This "cue like a cooking show" approach can leave silent space in your classes, allowing you to share words of wisdom without making the class feel crowded.

While many, many cueing principles follow this section, if you can grasp this one approach to cueing, you will dramatically improve your clarity and confidence when you teach. There are four clear components to delivering a yoga class: context, education, instructions, and atmosphere.

The method and desired results of each component differ, but together they yield a comprehensive understanding of what to do and how to do it. For this reason, we are going to look at these four components of delivering a class separately.

Journaling Activity

Do you remember a time when a teacher offered a cue that you could not understand? I remember once being told to "blossom my bottom open," and to this day, I am not certain I was doing it.

Not every cue will land for every person, but sometimes we need to refine our cues to achieve greater clarity for more people.

Context

When you flip a cookbook open to a certain recipe, authors will have often added a preamble as to why they included this recipe, what or who inspired them to develop it, or the recipe's heritage and cultural relevance. The information is not explicitly necessary to make the recipe, but it enriches the experience.

When you decide to teach a yoga class, you have a variety of pressures on you that can be difficult to balance. You have to deal with time constraints, various needs/abilities/challenges in the room, your own expectations of teaching, and your students' expectations. Whatever the limitations may be, we can alleviate some of them through conversational connection with students.

I like having people sit up for this conversation for a few reasons. Some benefits of beginning your class with a talk is that it provides an opportunity to form a personal connection with students, address any concerns that they have, and get information about participants. As mentioned earlier, how people feel about an activity impacts how that activity feels in their body. Students may feel more confident in movement if they feel connected to you beyond just the disembodied voice of a teacher starting the class.

There are some cueing elements that will be quite repetitive, and some that you will have to prepare before you teach. This component of teaching requires preparation each week, and perhaps the addition of a few notes before your teaching plan.

Here is a list of informative topics you may want to consider offering at the beginning of class:

- **Your name.** Offer your name and encourage folks to introduce themselves after class (though occasionally people tell me their names on the spot!).
- **Props required for class.** You could offer to retrieve the props or redistribute them if several people have lots of blocks and some people have none.
- **Inquiring if anyone is new to yoga.** If they are, congratulate them on their excellent decision while reassuring them that you are available and will keep an eye out for them.
- **Introduce a theme to the class.** Talk about some yoga philosophy, Ayurveda and seasonal practices, an anatomy/physiology tidbit, or share a story from your life that informs practice.
- **Clarify techniques or approaches.** Include this segment before the flow of class gets going.
- **Take requests.** This is optional—do this only if you are willing to work in a request that is appropriate to the class style and attendees, and you're able to sequence on the fly.

Some yogis like to share their upcoming workshops at the beginning of class, but I like to share this information at the end, when students are more likely to remember.

Asking About Injuries

Many teachers start class by asking, "Does anyone have an injury I should know about?" If you ask this question, you need to know what your response options will be and remember to stay within the scope of practice of a yoga teacher.

If someone does have an injury, rather than discussing their injury with the whole room, let them know you will come speak to them one-on-one. Set the rest of the class up in *Savasana* or another supported shape to begin class, and go over to the student's mat to find out more. Ask them if they have medical advice to practice yoga, and if they know how to modify positions or need some guidance as the class moves along.

Students seeing clinicians or therapists for specific injuries may have a higher knowledge of that joint and area than you do. Ask them what their injury means for movement practice, and if they cannot say, ask a few example questions, like "Can you bear weight on your hands? Can you lie on your belly?" They will get the point and may tell you more in a way that makes sense for providing options.

Education

A chef once told me there is a difference between a cookbook and a recipe book. Recipe books merely list out instructions for a variety of recipes, but a good cookbook teaches you how to develop your cooking methods. Cookbooks offer techniques that are helpful, as well as point out potential pitfalls to avoid, and offer you variations or substitutions that are appropriate within the framework of the recipe.

At the beginning of class, at a logical point after warm-up, or after a challenging sequence when yogis may appreciate a few moments to sit and listen, you can "workshop" some information. There is so much information worth conveying to yogis, but often it needs their full attention—music off, eyes and minds on the teacher. Use class opening or a break in a class to talk about...

- **Yoga postures or activities that are difficult to see.** Some poses are hard to demonstrate during the class no matter where you stand. If you discuss this in an upfront way, you can invite a student to demonstrate, or you can demonstrate how to set up different activities, including postures that are close to the ground or require supervision, like a headstand setup.

- **Prop use.** There are so many setup options, and while props are one size, yogis are many sizes. Those supported postures have a variety of ways they can be set up, and students may not be able to see their options from the back of the room. Demonstrate the various options, and then move around the room to assist people.

- **Anatomy/physiology lesson.** Maybe you want to clarify the difference between passive and active range, or you want to emphasize to students that conscious breathing is quite possibly the most important component of a yoga class. When people are moving, their concentration is committed to honing those new pathways of movement. If a lesson is worth learning, take a break for a couple of minutes to make it clear.

Instructions

Methods start to build a self-reliant repertoire, such that if you've done it enough times, you could cook a meal without a recipe. However, if the methods are not yet entrenched, if the content is new, or if we just need to be told what to do, the instructions must be laid out in a tested and proven sequence—the steps to achieving the desired results.

Instructions are the framework, foundation, and most critical element of teaching *yoga-asana* classes. Before you have enough mental energy to offer some inspiring details, you must be able to deliver classes that leave students feeling confident and refreshed. Before you can educate students on methods and subtleties, you need to accrue enough teaching time and wisdom to have observations to impart.

Cues that translate into movements and engagement are particularly crucial because there is nothing descriptive about yoga pose names. We may mistakenly believe that to be a valuable teacher, we must be unique, but if novelty were the most reliable indicator of good teaching, many other successful teachers and I would be out of jobs.

The following principles of cueing students through activities will work for you, along with some practice and observation. They will help you develop your personal cueing repertoire, one that you can refine over your career, rather than prescriptively describing one way to cue a posture or activity.

Cue Embodiment Instead of Postures (the "Simon says" Rule)

Teaching people how to *embody* rather than simply saying pose names is critical for several reasons.

First of all, you are teaching. Teaching is explaining. There is nothing explanatory about the words "Half Moon," so teaching this pose requires you to provide instructions for people to get there. Once they are mostly there, you can refine for greater understanding and success.

Second, there are too many movement exercises we teach that are not yoga postures with names. We need to articulate movements as clearly as possible so that we can diversify our activities and sequences and offer people a rich, efficient movement experience.

Demonstrating is not a substitute for honing your communication skills. The nuances of an embodiment cannot be perceived through casual observation while simultaneously practicing, so proper cueing and timely, skillful demonstrating are best. These examples will help illustrate what good cueing might look like.

- Example 1: From Tabletop pose, step your left foot back and put your heel down, parallel to the short end of your mat, as if you were going into Warrior II *(Virabhadrasana II)*. Swing your right shin behind you like a kickstand, and lift your left arm to the ceiling as you turn your torso upward to the left. Circle your left arm over your head to arrive in a variation of *Parighasana*, Gate pose.
- Example 2: Lying on your back, bend your knees and keep some space between your feet. Your hips, knees

and feet line up. Bring your arms down by your sides, make fists, and bend your elbows so your fists point to the ceiling, sort of like robot arms. Keep your elbows close to you. Press firmly into your feet and roll your spine up off the mat, starting from the tailbone and up to the top of the spine. Lift as high as you can. Beginning at the top of your spine near your shoulders, roll your spine back down to the mat. Continue rolling up and down, into and out of Bridge pose.

- Example 3: As you stand on your right foot with your hands on your hips, lift your left knee as high into your chest as you can. Spread your toes, draw your navel in toward your spine, and try to bring your chest evenly back over your pelvis so that you're leaning toward the back of the room. If it's going well, reach your hands to the ceiling and put a lot of lift in your chest, while keeping your lower belly strong. This variation of Tree pose is super strengthening, and now we're going to add some movement...

Keep It Simple

As a teacher, especially in drop-in yoga studios, where we happily accommodate the continuous inflow of yoga novices, you compete with a long list of distractions and potential confusion. How students receive instructions depends dramatically on their context: language(s) spoken, learning preferences, body awareness, yoga experience, stress levels, life events, etc.

Journaling Activity

1. Without using pose names, write the cues for a Sun Salutation, or a variation that you teach.
2. Design a mini-sequence of four postures that you enjoy linked together, like Warrior II → Extended Side Angle → Triangle → Half Moon. Write the cues for this sequence; again, without using pose names.
3. Think of a mini-sequence of exercises that do not have specific pose names. Write cues for these movements and transitions.

Note: Write these in pencil or type them up, as we'll want to be able to edit them soon!

Listening may seem simple—your ears register sounds that the brain interprets, and we respond in thought or action—when in reality, the process is much more complicated, given that you are competing with external and internal distractions. Processing words into understanding requires mental energy; translating audio signs (words) into kinesthetic expression (movement) requires even more.

Keeping it simple includes using the present, active tense and few words (where possible). For example, "Do this," rather than "And now you are going to do this."

- Example 1 (Balancing core strength): Set yourself up on hands and knees. Reach your right arm forward and your left leg back. Draw your lower belly in so your lower back is still. Look calmly at the ground as you build a little heat.

- Example 2 (*Nadi Shodhana Pranayama*): Make a peace sign and bring those fingers together. Put them on your forehead. Cover your right nostril with your thumb. Breathe out your left nostril. Breathe in your left nostril. Cover your left nostril with your remaining fingers and hold your nose closed. Pause. Now release your thumb and exhale out your right nostril. Inhale through your right nostril. Cover with your thumb again and pause before exhaling out your left nostril. Continue alternating breath between your nostrils.

Cue From the Student's Perspective

Have you ever had a teacher say something like, "Turn over here and then..." but they are nowhere to be seen? Or the teacher offers you some options within a posture, but they are only understandable if you break position to stand up and look at the teacher demonstrating?

If you cue from the *student's* perspective, they do not need to look at you as much. This means that you are free to walk around and observe your class, and, most importantly, the students get to have an improved internal experience through more opportunity to practice with closed eyes.

- Example 1: Move your knees closer to your hands.

If people knew where their hips were, they would put their knees under them. If you are telling students to line their hands up under their shoulders, their knees under their hips, or their ribs over their pelvis and they are not doing the actions correctly, it means they cannot tell where they are in space. Instead, use landmarks that make more sense to them. For example, if a student's Tabletop pose is too elongated, ask them to bring their knees closer to their *hands*, which are a more visual landmark.

- Example 2: Turn to face the stone wall in a wide-legged stance.

You can use the room you are in to help cue! Lots of studios have landmarks in the room, like plants, platforms, clocks, prop walls, painted walls, walls with the door you came through, etc., that you can use to direct people. If you set up a yoga studio or teaching space, consider having at least one colored wall to orient students, and then a few defining features to assist your teaching. You can then cue "toward the orange wall," or "toward the prayer flags."

Students are probably practicing on a yoga mat, so the corners, short sides, and long sides of their mats are also good landmarks. If you had students place their blocks on either side of the front of their mat at the beginning of class, those become great landmarks too.

- Example 3 (in Downward-facing Dog): Press the tops of your thighs back a bit and draw your lower belly in, as if you were wearing a belt and wanted to show more of it to the floor. With your lower belly engaged, it should feel like you're helping your belt do its job.

Most people know what wearing a belt is like, but they may not know what "engage your abdominal muscles in Downward-facing Dog" is like. We can look for creative ways that draw on people's experiences to help them understand some helpful engagements that will improve their practice.

Cue for Building Boundaries and Targeted Engagement

Many people think they are doing a posture optimally, even when, as the teacher, you can see that certain joints are not optimally relaxed, are contracting, or seem to be doing their own thing entirely.

For example, you are teaching hip circles from Tabletop position, with one leg circling. Your students will naturally lean away from the side they are working.

Tell the students what is happening so that they take notice of it, and then offer helpful advice from their perspective.

- Example 1 (Hip circles in Tabletop): You're leaning to the left, so bring your spine back to center, which will feel like a lot more effort on your right side. Spread your toes so your right leg is active, and as you lift your shoulders off your arms a bit, press your outer left hip back a bit and keep it there.
- Example 2 (Plank pose with knees down): For integrity, you may need to place your knees on the ground, where you can also do a more targeted approach to engaging abdominal muscles by feeling like your hands and knees are squeezing toward each other.

Use the Second Person Perspective/Associate the Yogi to Their Body

The first person perspective consists of "I" statements, as in, "I hope there are some cookies left!" The third person perspective is the omniscient voice that is typically found in fiction, as in, "Kathryn went to the cupboard looking for cookies."

Using the second person perspective is rare, unless we are giving instructions. It consists of "you" statements, as in, "You will find no cookies in the cupboard, Kathryn." When we teach our classes, use the second person perspective to describe the practice to our students.

This may seem stuffy, but stay with me.

We all consume a lot of media, and one of the insidious effects of media exposure is the compartmentalization of the self. Instead of seeing ourselves as holistic beings of a body-mind experience, we parcel ourselves off into various works-in-progress: *My mind is too chaotic, so I must do meditation for it, but my bum is too big, so I must run to make it smaller,* or *My arms are too weak, so I must do Sun Salutations to make them stronger.*

Our yoga practice can help us discern the difference between uncomfortable experiences and activities that are possibly injurious. We can help people cultivate their own body intuition by using the second person perspective in our teaching. This approach also enhances feelings of personal connection between student and teacher. Students often say that my classes feel like a conversation, and I think that this particular cueing principle creates that atmosphere of dialogue.

- Example 1: Your hand, rather than "that hand."
- Example 2: Close your eyes. Now that you've finessed the posture, simply be in the posture. Observe what it's like to breathe your breath in this shape, fully immersed in the present moment, rooted down into your feet, connected at your center, and reaching up through your arms.

This is one of the many gifts of yoga: cultivating a holistic experience of body. Let your students lay claim to their body-minds as whole, functioning beings, and cue with the second person perspective.

Journaling Activity

Return to the write-ups you did for the first principle, "Cue Embodiment Instead of Postures" (the one where you wrote out the cues for various mini-sequences) and see if they could be edited to exchange disembodied cues ("that hand") for more personal cues ("your hand").

Teach the "Brown rice version"...and Then Add Toppings

Rice bowls need rice as a foundation of the dish by definition, so leave details and nuances of embodiment and expression for after building the foundation of a pose.

- Example 1 (Warrior I): Step your right foot between your hands. Put your back heel down. Check that your feet are on separate tracks, and your back foot is sort of pointing forward. Stand up and reach your arms up. As you lunge into your front leg, your back leg stays straight.
- Example 2 (Headstand): Step down onto your forearms and measure the distance between your arms by holding your hands to your biceps. Keep your elbows exactly where they are, release your biceps, and interlace your fingers. Start pressing your forearms down as you lift your knees up.
- Example 3 (Reclined Bicycle): Slowly mimic an upside-down bicycle ride and turn up the resistance. Some of you are speeding in the slow lane—slow it down. Put 10–20 inches of space between your legs, and explore space as your hips, knees, and ankles bend and lengthen.

...Rice Bowl Topping Examples

Clear instructions for successful movement are not as interesting or sexy as the artistic cues ("Now let's marinate here for a minute..."), but they are essential.

There are so many nuances to movement and alignment, and teachers must consistently refine how we offer descriptions. These examples build on the previous foundations.

- Example 1, Warrior I *(Virabhadrasana I)*: Press down through your back heel and evenly wrap the muscles of your back leg forward. Your heel centers anchor, but also actively spread the muscles of your feet like you were trying to fill out Birkenstocks. Pull the front points of your pelvis toward each other and up a little bit.

- Example 2, Headstand (*Sirsasana*): Press downward through your headstand foundation, and walk your feet closer to your elbows. Actively lift your hips up as much as you press your arms down.
- Example 3, Reclined Bicycle: You may experiment with going higher toward the ceiling and lower toward the ground (go higher toward the ceiling if you feel a pull in your lower back). Have you ever been too lazy to pet the dog with your hand, so you do it with your foot? Bring that quality to the movement.

Use Cues Drawn From Real Life

In Warrior II *(Virabhadrasana II)*, yogis will often chase their front hand and lean forward in the posture. Teachers will often say "Bring your ribs back over your pelvis," and this works for some people, but not others. One day, I asked students to "belly dance their ribs" back over their pelvis, and it worked! Even though I think very few of them had actually ever tried belly dancing...

Other examples that have worked for me are:

- Runner's Lunge: Lean forward like someone shot you out of a cannon.
- Seated Twist/Half Lord of the Fishes (*Ardha Matsyendrasana)*: Some of you are leaning back like you're trying to talk to someone in the seat behind you, so draw your ribs forward so you are more situated over your pelvis.

- Thread the Needle *(Parsva Balasana,* flow variation): You are reaching up really enthusiastically, like you are close to getting a coin out of the couch!
- Chair *(Utkatasana)*: Pressing down through your heels, find the muscles that would hop you backwards, but stay still.

Begin Pose Options With the Accessible, and Then Add Challenges

Let us resist using a few phrases around options like "The next level of this pose is…" or "The goal of this pose is to eventually…" or "For the advanced version…."

First of all, what is an advanced yoga posture? There are people who come to the yoga mat and, through genetically-gifted flexibility or a dance career, can execute "advanced" yoga postures their first time trying them. Similarly, lots of people can sit still on the outside, but are freaking out and feeding their distracted minds on the inside. Appearances are deceiving, and purely aesthetic experiences of yoga are superficial.

We are trying to evolve the exchange of how it *looks* for how it *feels*. What it looks like should matter less, and so we should avoid cues that imply one version is superior or more advanced than another.

Each variation has its own benefits worth exploring in the service of a well-rounded practice. Here are a few ways we can work with offering options, while keeping our language less competitive.

- Example 1 (Dolphin toward Forearm Balance): Place your forearms on the ground, keeping your wrists in line with your elbows—a block between the hands can help us with shoulder engagement here. Curl your toes under and lift your hips up. Walk your feet closer than you want to. Pick up your right leg and—keeping it very straight—reach your hips and your leg up to the ceiling. Keep this leg straight. If you like, bend your supporting leg and take light hops with quiet landings. If you like, slow down your attempts to begin lifting both legs toward forearm balance.

- Example 2 (Half Moon): While standing on your right foot with your left leg lifted, hold a block under your right hand and put your left hand on your left hip. Press out through your left heel, straighten your right leg and broaden across your pelvis. Broaden and lengthen your chest, starting to lift it upward, more in line with your pelvis. You may want to reach your left arm to the ceiling. You may want to take your right hand off the block, and put a big reach between your arms. If you're feeling sassy, put your right hand on your heart.

Use Positive, Inclusive Phrasing

Many of us develop some deeply negative self-talk about our abilities because we obsess over things we are not "supposed" to do in our lives. The antidote is to limit the number of times we tell our students what they're not going to do, and instead focus on what we are going to do.

To come back to our recipe analogy, rarely does a recipe read, "Do not put fennel in this recipe instead of the cinnamon." That recipe would instead simply say, "Mix in 1 teaspoon of cinnamon." In yoga, this translates to using positive instructions:

- Example: Instead of "Don't put your knee down," instruct students to "Put your back heel down, and keep your knee up."

You may be thinking, surely this is not possible, or it is artificially cheerful. I know that it is possible with effort, and would encourage you to work toward mostly positive phrasing. Sometimes, however, you do need to clarify the difference between what you may think is right and what is actually desirable—recipes do this all the time!

Telling people what not to do doesn't tell them what they should be doing. Read my example below to clarify how you can do that gently and informatively.

- Example: In *Utthan Pristhasana*/Lizard pose, you will be tempted to round your upper back and get really drawn into what is happening in your hips. Try to lengthen your mid-back instead, and keep lifting your ribs forward off your waistline and broaden across your collarbone. Your head and neck can look forward or at the ground, but lengthen the space between your earlobes and shoulders. The demanding hip extension in our back leg and flexion in our front hip makes this hard work. Keep strengthening your upper back through lengthening, as you press down under your front foot and straighten through your back leg.

Journaling Activity

Journal about a time when a teacher's description of different experiences caught your attention during class. It could be something you wanted to integrate into your own teaching, or something you'd prefer not to integrate.

What are some ways you can express exploration of options without describing them as advanced or implying levels of development?

Human Embodiment is Diverse

Large cities and the online yoga world often offer classes for various aspects of the embodied human experiences. There are yoga classes for ages at both ends of the spectrum (kids yoga and yoga for seniors). There are classes for people with disabilities, particular health conditions, and navigating difficult transitions or personal history.

Niche-specific classes (like "Yoga for Seniors", "Parent and Baby Yoga" and "BIPOC Yoga") speak to the importance of community that reflects your embodied experience, and the healing capacity for meaning-making and practice in specific groups.

Language is a practice of awareness for yogis. In community classes open "to everyone," this requires consideration for how our language habits celebrate the diversity of human embodiment. While a variety of aspects of the human embodiment experience, including gender, are sources of joy and expression for each of us, they can also be sources of pain.

Yoga is a practice premised on the realization of a universal Self or Truth, and that Self exists beyond gender. We can use language that evokes universal aspects of embodiment to promote inclusivity in the studio.

For example...

- My preferred greeting for a group is "Hello yogis." Buddhist groups often use "yogis" to refer to participants because it is gender-neutral. "Hello folks!" works nicely, too. "Hello bright souls" is also lovely.
- Refer to student by their names. Instead of saying, "you two boys partner up!" You can say "Daud and Mike, you two can partner up!" In any circumstance, learning your students' names is a powerful reminder to them that they matter and that you care about them.
- If you are working in a demonstration with a student and you do not know their preferred pronouns, you can use their name or the neutral pronoun of "they". If Kay is demonstrating for you, you could say, "look at Kay's hand placement – see how they have it holding their shin?"
- Use common body parts when you're referring to specific areas of the body. If you're struggling to describe

certain areas of the body, brainstorm outside of class time. For example, you can describe "turning the upper portion of your chest to the left", or you can also use "heartspace" or "pectoral muscles," if you think your class knows where those muscles are!

- When using cues drawn from real life, resist the urge to qualify the cue with a gender context. I often cue "the part of your foot where the weight in a high heeled shoe would go", because students sometimes cannot tell where "the ball" of the foot is. There's no need to add anything about who wears high-heeled shoes.

- Speak to your own experience in *dharma* talks or shares. As we discussed at the beginning of the book, you *should* bring your life forward into your practice. There is no yoga without your life, but our lives are both unique and common. I will often speak to my experience of motherhood, but I root the talk in my experience and then bridge it to the more universal aspects of experience I'm using it to illustrate. (Like the desire for good sleep!)

I've been in classes where teachers use an exclusive cue and then they try to rationalize it as they go along. For example, telling students to use self-massage balls near where their bra strap should be, and then going on about who wears bras and how other people can imagine where it is, etc. I think this happens because they realized the cue was exclusive, unnecessary or inappropriate, and then their anxiety mounted, causing them to continue on.

Every yoga teacher and spiritual facilitator regrets a cue or two. Teaching yoga is a public speaking gig, and the momentum and complexity of teaching have carried an unskillful phrase from many tongues. Rather than digging the anxiety hole deeper while teaching, gather yourself, take a breath, and keep teaching.

Those feelings of anxiety are not helpful at the moment, but they will direct you toward a more skillful awareness of language in the future. As you reflect on your teaching and what you may choose to do differently, practice self-compassion with yourself by acknowledging what you've learned and move forward.

Reflection and Atmosphere

Finally, many cookbook authors want you to feel inspired and invigorated by their recipes. They want you to explore the process creatively. There may be a bullet list of ways you could change the recipe (different variations), or a beautiful photo of the final dish once complete. Maybe they offer suggestions for how you could serve it...though I've always wondered about who cleans up the scattered ingredients from those photo shoots...

A yoga class is a mixture of artistry and science, and here are some of the elements that may feel artistic, but, rest assured, a graduate student somewhere is researching the benefits.

Make Space for Silence

Whether you teach to tabla drum beats and sitar or folksy covers of Coldplay, create space for silence in your classes. We all experience elective noise—music, conversations, television, etc.—but we also experience pervasive non-elective noise from driving, being in the community, and the hum of machines.

A student with a traumatic brain injury once asked me if my silent retreat was completely silent. When I asked her to clarify, she gestured to a tea warmer and said, "I hear all of that as foreground noise. My brain can't differentiate between background and foreground anymore. Everything is noise."

While that may be a specific example, most of us cannot appreciate to what degree our world is noise-saturated.

Music can play a role in your classes, but Ayurveda says silence is necessary for digestion. From the Ayurvedic perspective, you consume *prana* (vital life force) through all five of your senses: sight, taste, touch, sound, and smell. Through the Western lens, we think of digestion as purely calorie- and taste-based—food comes in, we extract what we need, and eliminate the waste.

Ayurveda says that the impressions you consume through your senses also need to be digested, otherwise they result in an accumulation of "the undigested" (*ama*, sometimes translated as toxicity), and this can cause us to feel unwell.

For optimal wellness, we must take breaks from our senses (*pratyahara*) and digest those impressions.

Offer Balanced Encouragement

Sometimes you need to be encouraging, and sometimes you need to clarify the activity of the movement. Do both with a certain amount of steadiness to your voice. We want to bring the enthusiasm, but encouraging too much extroverted energy is contrary to the intention of cultivating an evenness of energy.

You also want to offer authentic praise for teaching moments, because sometimes excessive praise for simple things can backfire. I once heard from a studio owner that she'd received a comment card reading, "I don't want to be praised for making my way to hands and knees."

Diversify the reasons you praise your students. If we only praise physical performance, we solidify it as the most important aspect of practice. Remember to praise "great focus", "beautiful smiles", "warm energy", etc.

Compassionately Remind Students When They're Distracted

Sometimes students are distracted, and you want to invite them back into their practice. There are lots of things you could say, but we want to be helpful, not angry that they're not listening. Getting distracted is a part of the practice; returning to attention is equally part of the practice.

Choose a Tone That Builds Atmosphere and Clarity

When guiding *Savasana*, your voice will be softer and soothing. If you are encouraging students who are doing a heating exercise, your tone will be empowering and encouraging. Your volume, tone, pitch, inflection, and words should all be in the service of your students' success.

For example, when I ask students to tiptoe to the front of the mat and lift their hips the whole way, I chirp "Hips up! Hips up! Hips up!" several times, with some pep to convey the continuity.

If your cues are toward movement, your voice can move up for the upward moving cues, and down with the downward moving cues. These subtleties are enormously effective at conveying nuance.

Try it! A good example is dragging out the vowel sounds in "slow" or "big" when cueing a repetitive movement—try it and let me know how it goes.

Activity

Jot down five movements or postures of different energy levels that you often teach. Practice cueing them, and as you cue, experiment with your voice to enhance the cue's message. For example, you may stretch out a vowel in a word to promote lingering.

Remember, language and movement are radically different - enhancing your message in the service of clarity is kind!

Savasana and Closing Classes

IN THE SAME WAY that it is lovely to linger at a table with conversation after a good meal, it is good to linger and digest after a good yoga practice. A *Savasana* and gentle class closing could look like this kind of flow.

Invite students into *Savasana*: Remind yogis that they can put on socks and sweaters, reach for props, and take their time to settle in. Count on 2–3 minutes for yogis to get settled here.

Offer seated meditation or a supported, integrative yoga shape: While seated meditation is not a superior practice to *Savasana*, it can be helpful for yogis who are not comfortable lying on the ground because of a body ache, sinus congestion, or who struggle with the mental pressures of laying prone. You can invite them to sit upright for their meditation, supported by a *zafu*, a block and blanket, or up against a wall.

Remind students how to use props for restful support: Offer instructions to yogis who are new to the practice, who have only practiced in hot yoga spaces, or those without soft props. They may need to know that bolsters go under their kneecaps (or the bottom of their thigh bones) and support the lower back. A blanket laid over the body can keep us warm, but even a folded blanket over the chest or lower abdomen can lend a sense of grounding.

Let students know if you are closing class with sitting upright and chanting: Some studios have their teachers leave students in *Savasana* without coming upright to sit. Let students know if deciding the length of *Savasana* is up to them and you will be leaving the room, or if you will be present for the duration and will close the practice in community. I tell the room, "The next time you hear my voice, it will be to begin the closing of class, which we do seated, together. This way, you do not need to worry about how long you should stay for *Savasana*. Enjoy this time."

Circle back to the class theme: If it is appropriate, revisit the class theme as a realized outcome of your practice.

Remind yogis that bringing awareness back is the practice: This is another lesson that you may feel is repetitive, but there may be someone in the room who needs this reminder to be gentle with themselves and the nature of their minds. Remind yogis that in the gentle, compassionate way you would redirect a child away from an undesirable distraction to the task at hand, you should reorient your mind.

Be quiet. Teachers often ask me what I do during *Savasana*, and my answer is that it depends on the class. If I have someone in class who may be experiencing mental distress and keeps their eyes open during *Savasana*, I calmly keep my eyes open and focus on a long breath practice (*Dirgha Pranayama*). Sometimes I silently recite *mantra*, and sometimes I do single-nostril breathing without the *mudra* (*Anuloma Viloma*). Sometimes I simply sit and think positive affirmations, or watch my thoughts bubble along. Paying attention and being able to respond, if needed, is the responsibility of the teacher.

Offer a reading: Select one that has been carefully chosen and pre-reviewed. Whether it is a song, poem, or passage, whatever you share in a yoga class should be listened to or read through *entirely* before sharing it with students. You never know if a song takes a dramatic turn or a poem includes an element too disturbing to share unless you review the whole song/reading.

Here is the script for how I close my classes...

Stay relaxed exactly as you are...closing with a reading from Mary Oliver entitled Wild Geese. *(Do the reading, and pause for absorption.)*

Begin to deepen your breath.

Reintroduce little movements that speak to you.

You may want to stretch long, and you may want to tuck in. You may want to roll to one side. You are welcome to do both on the way back to seated.

There is no hurry, and when you return to seated, connect your palms and connect your thumbs and your heart.

We'll close with two breaths, the second is the sound of OM.

Take a deep breath in, and gently let it go. Breathing in to chant, OM.

Thank you so much for your practice; it's a privilege to teach.

Finally, you can thank people again for their curiosity, enthusiasm, gentleness—whatever it is that speaks to you. Remind them that they can find you for your upcoming workshop or retreat, and that you're happy to answer any questions they may have.

Responsible Encouragement

Part of teaching yoga is offering students feedback and encouragement. We are offering feedback based on the average performance in the room, and only want to offer what is helpful. To be skillful in our application of encouragement, we can consider the timing, content, and culture of feedback.

Culture
Modern Western yoga culture shares territory with fitness culture. Yes, exercise is beneficial, but exercise culture can pro-

mote feelings of never being "good enough," body dysmorphia, and perfectionism.

Fitness culture relies on maxims like "just do it" and "leaving it all on the floor," but in yoga, we strive for a more nuanced understanding of effort. "Leaving it all on the floor" assumes that you have no partner, children, aging parents, or pets to care for, and the health and finances to bounce back from exhaustion.

Ayurveda, yoga's sister science, suggests that our exercise should only facilitate sweating to 50% of our capacity, leaving us feeling revitalized and refreshed. Students can control the intensity of their practice with encouragement from us, but only if we shape a class culture informed by self-compassion, cultivating our bodymind intuition, and not relying on teachers to dictate when breaks are appropriate.

Here are some sentiments you can share that will help you do that in your classes.

> *Please remember that we are here to cultivate compassionate discipline, not desperation. If you feel yourself spiraling in inner distraction, consider taking a break from the practice.*

> *I'm going to count down the rest of this activity, so you know when it ends.*

> *This is a practice premised on cultivating an inner compass to direct our actions and our peacefulness. Please take a moment to acknowledge that you are both the compass and the explorer—I'm just the tour guide. All offerings are optional.*

Internally distracting yourself or "bearing with it" may be signs that we need to take a break, and some coping mechanisms are counterproductive to your goals. Work with yourself, not against yourself, and take a steady, compassionate approach to practice.

Beginning of Class

Whenever a student is in their first yoga class, meditation workshop, or retreat, I typically smile and congratulate them on their good decision. Then I usually say that these practices can be difficult sometimes, but life seems to be more difficult without them.

At the beginning of class, you may want to share something that acknowledges both the benefits of practice and some of the challenges.

Take a moment to express gratitude to yourself and all the people who are helping you be here today.

One of my favorite understandings of yoga is making space—you made space in your budget and calendar to be here, you're making space in the room with your mat, and we will make space in the bodymind with practice. Thank yourself for making space today.

Sometimes the most difficult part of practice is beginning. Acknowledge your commitment and take a deep breath into your heart space.

Whatever is happening in your life that is outside your control, your presence here acknowledges that challenges may not be so turbulent or difficult if you take some time out.

During Class

Teaching movement, stillness, or breath requires offering instructions, allowing the students to "do the thing," and perhaps providing feedback along the way.

If they are "doing the thing" and you observe that their method and energy is just fine, perhaps offer no feedback. The older I get, the more I hear from students about how much they needed that quiet time in their practice.

If you observe that it is appropriate to offer some feedback or encouragement, remember that some people need permission to stop, and some people benefit from the encouragement to continue. How do we strike a balance between these needs? Consider the following suggestions.

We're exploring how to do difficult things with grace. Sometimes the practice of grace looks like taking a break, and sometimes it's continuing with the activity with less gripping.

We're building calm and compassionate strength and discipline.

Yes! I can see you integrating the methods really well.

Feeling that one expression of a posture is superior in healthfulness is a misunderstanding of how bodies work. Your expression is healthful, beneficial, and perfect.

Before we try that again, let's get clear and present so that our effort is calm.

Some bits of great parenting advice also apply beautifully to teaching yoga, such as "Focus less on the desired outcome, and more on the effort." You could tell your class the following sentiment:

I can see you're focusing with determination while remaining gentle in your energy. Well done.

Ending Class

Conclusions are difficult, but ending your class on time with a few words of gratitude is all you need to do.

You were so present in our practice today, thank you.

Thank you for being here with me to cultivate our skillfulness.

Thank you for your practice; it's a privilege to teach. OM, Shanti, peace.

Demonstrating

BEFORE SOMEONE BEGINS A yoga program, they likely have a vague expectation of what will happen in a class, given yoga's popularity in pop culture and media. This expectation of class likely includes the teacher "doing the yoga" in perfect synchronicity with the students.

If you practice yoga for even a short time, you know that perfect synchronicity throughout a class is impossible, and that teachers take varying approaches to demonstrating during class.

I advocate for using demonstrating discerningly, as a tool rather than a rule. There are several benefits to the teaching-off-the-mat approach, but first, why demonstrate in the first place?

Yoga's history as "yoga"—the movement/exercise activity that transpires on a rectangular mat—is contested, non-linear, and it was never a foregone conclusion that *yoga-asana* would be the primary adopted practice of the yogic system. As recently depicted in the popular (and vastly watchable) Netflix documentary, *Wild Wild Country,* there was an appetite for Indian metaphysics and guru-culture in the West throughout the 1960s and 1970s. Meditation, *yoga-asana*, and spiritual practices outside Western organized religion had evolved from curiosities to something one could actually participate in. That is a radical shift in culture, as India has a long history of yoga being for both householders and renunciates, but it was a fringe, even frightening, practice elsewhere.

During this era of change, there was a dramatic cultural shift driven by an interest in inner inquiry and political activism. Yoga could have continued to be a radical activity, but it eventually merged with fitness culture and shifted its emphasis toward physical healthfulness and achieving an idealized body.[39]

As the interest in consciousness-raising movements waned, the 1980s arrived, with a more extroverted popular culture driven by consumerism and individual signs of success over collective consciousness-raising. Bodybuilding and gym culture became popularized, and working out at home grew more common, with women taking fitness cues from Jane Fonda.[40] Workouts could be done in front of the television and would not interrupt the domestic duties of housewives. (I want to note that Jane Fonda is not only a former exercise video mogul, but also a longtime activist with five decades of experience who has been arrested five times for her eco-activism event, Fire Drill Fridays. Just in case you were worried that it had to be a choice between activist *or* fitness enthusiast!).

Over the latter half of the 20th century, BKS Iyengar and Sri Pattabhi Jois came to America to promote their schools of yoga. They were both students to Tirumalai (TKV) Krishnam-acharya, who is considered the most influential innovator of modern yoga.

Krishnamacharya popularized yoga within India before his students left for the West, and he blended his knowledge of yoga with the gymnastics-based approach to fitness educa-tion implemented through British colonial rule. Krishnamacha-rya, like many yoga figures, was complex and troubling—he was abusive toward his students, but also a renowned healer and scholar.

His students, Jois and Iyengar, may have increased the ath-leticism of the practice to appeal more to the layperson, who was increasingly more concerned with physical fitness than a spiritual practice. Yoga scholar Mark Singleton also argues that such teachers, particularly Iyengar in his popular text *Light on Yoga*, insist that yoga postures are more than simply gymnas-tics, but never truly qualify why they are inherently more spiri-tual than gymnastics.[41]

(Sri Pattabhi Jois has also been celebrated as a central fig-ure in modern yoga. However, his reputation is being posthu-mously revised, as many of his female former students have come forward to share their experience of sexual assault dur-ing Jois's hands-on adjustments.)[42]

Demonstrating and hands-on adjustments are sometimes juxtaposed as two approaches to teaching, but you can en-tirely leave out hands-on in your teaching and still need to refine how you demonstrate and cue your classes. Demon-strating should always accompany a strong effort to express instructions from the students' point of view for clarity and to promote their movement intuition.

There is little historical evidence from which we can draw on, but I believe that the rolled out mat at the front of the room for a teacher to demonstrate on is a specific result of the collision of Iyengar and Jois's emphasis on *asana* (Jois had a famous refrain: "99% practice and 1% theory") and the ripeness of fitness culture that was emerging in the 1980s. Like yoga teachers, fitness instructors make a low wage, and often work without job security and benefits—many have full-time jobs supplemented by teaching fitness (why not do what you were going to do anyway, but get a free gym membership out of it?).

Exercise is an essential component for wellness, and it is the reason that yoga is thriving. Spirituality and ethical precepts are not a precondition for practicing yoga, and if they were, I would not be writing this book, as I would have chosen the Hare Krishna—they have tambourines. We must acknowledge the maxim *to meet the student where they are,* and that if their interest in practice is hamstring-stretching and core work, that is a good practice.

However, allow me to pick up where Iyengar left off, and point out that there are some key differences (even in the qualities and characteristics of yogic exercise as compared to a fitness exercise) that we may want to explore before we talk about the specifics of demonstrating.

Group exercise classes have an element of extroversion to them; yet, yoga is a practice that helps us explore our interior life. Group exercise classes often rely on external distractions—loud music, shouted encouragement, etc.—and keep you visually engaged (practicality is at play here too; no one recommends grapevining with your eyes closed).

The fitness room set up—instructor at front and all participants facing them—creates an "all eyes on me" atmosphere. Modern Western yoga culture adopted the same set up, and it keeps a lot of teachers and students stuck in some deeply held patterns. If we want to de-emphasize a particular aesthetic in yoga and emphasize inner transformation, we have to consider how we use demonstrating thoughtfully.

Do students need to watch the teacher in a yoga class?

Sometimes you need to demonstrate, but not as frequently as you may think necessary. As a yoga participant, even if you do not know the term for the activity and have never done it before, you can approximate what other people in the room are doing. Demonstrating works best if everyone is upright and knows where the teacher is in the room.

As a yoga teacher, you have to move around the room to be in front of, or in the midst of, your students for effective demonstrating. For example, if you wanted to add arm movements into a Goddess pose foundation, you would have to move to the side of the room that the students are facing. If there are a lot of people in the room, you may want to simply stand to only demonstrate the arm movement so that you're taller than everyone and the people in the back can see what you're doing.

If students are on their hands and knees, you may want to get among them near the front of the room, so that the few people near you "get it" and then understanding and execution ripples outward from the center.

There are limitations to what demonstrating teaches. Students can approximate embodiment, but they need more specific instruction on how to engage, where to relax, and the other subtleties they are trying to discern. Muscular engagement is not evident from looking at someone else, not to mention the impossibility of simultaneously observing for detail. For example, if you step yourself into Warrior II, some teachers say to push the feet down and away from each other, while others say to draw them toward each other—you could never know just from looking.

That means that I could just do the posture and then cue what I'm doing, right?

Sure, you could, but what if students are already doing 90% of the pose correctly, or need fewer of your cues? A key takeaway from this book would be to *increase the silence in your classes and practice and observe what is happening in the room.* Many teachers who only demonstrate their classes chatter through their postures—without observing what is happening in the room in front of you, you are compelled to say everything that may be necessary/helpful. If your students are already doing the thing, then say less and give them blissful silence. You are there to teach, they are there to practice.

Yoga is changing.

There are many yoga postures and activities where students cannot see your demonstration. However the yoga mats are arranged, any activities done lying prone on the back or supine on the front are not going to be viewable. If you rely on students seeing you to convey your teachings, they will be confused when they are doing anything other than standing and looking forward.

Also, if you are on the ground demonstrating, you will not be able to see the students who need your help because they are misinterpreting your cues. Getting up and moving around the room makes you available to help students who need individual guidance into or out of a position.

There are also less obvious benefits to cutting down on demonstrations when cueing your classes. Sustaining an injury, which is a real threat to anyone who teaches regularly, is less likely. I once crossed paths in the teachers' room with another yogi who was heading to the emergency room ahead of a flight because she badly pulled a muscle in class. Other teachers develop chronic imbalances from inattentive demonstrating or always demonstrating the first side and rarely the second side.

If you are demonstrating to "sneak in" some yoga postures for yourself, you need to make more space for personal practice, even perhaps teaching less. Stealing (*steya*) snippets of practice for your physical well-being does not feel right for the spirit. There is no good karma to achieve from teaching a practice that you do not do! The teachers who stick with teaching long-term always survive the eventual imbalance of teaching/ practice ratios by recommitting to their practice.

Atmosphere matters, and your voice shapes the atmosphere.

Planking and public speaking do not improve each other. I sound a lot less calm and confident when I speak while exerting myself through exercise. The quality of your voice will be more steady and richer if you are standing or sitting. If you are exercising on the mat along with your students, that effort shows up in your voice.

Ask yourself, what atmosphere are you trying to create? While students may not be able to articulate that there is a connection between the limited demonstrating I do and the quality of my voice, they know the latter is something they find appealing.

When teacher trainees in continuing education workshops say to me that their students rely on them to demonstrate, I remind them that their students only depend on them to show the postures because that is the precedent. Lessening the frequency of demonstrating by degrees will gradually change students' expectations and build everyone's confidence.

Are there any good times to demonstrate?

If you are going to reduce your demonstration, the best times to pare down are during activities close to the ground. One of the times it makes sense to keep some demonstrating included is during seated portions of class. There are a lot of excellent, accessible activities done from a seated position that you can lead, while smiling at your students in connected practice.

Another good time to offer a demonstration is when there is widespread misunderstanding in the room, you are offering something new that requires additional instruction, or you are asking everyone to observe how you set up props.

You could also demonstrate at the beginning of class to prepare students for a planned activity. This is a helpful approach because students will be able to see you, or can move to see you better.

When I am teaching a props setup, I use one student and set them up with different options (leaving them in the one they want) and then offer help to the room. Here are the cues that I use after demonstrating a supported backbend setup.

- Whichever option you have chosen, your bum should be on the ground and able to relax.
- If your bum is floating, we may want to put a blanket underneath it.
- Your legs could be crossed—lower backs like that—and extended, or knees can be bent and touching.
- Your arms could be by your sides, on your heart and belly, or overhead.
- You could also let your arms bend and float out at your sides, or join fingers overhead. You could then crawl your fingers toward your elbows.
- If you need me to double check the setup, that is why I am here—the major benefit of practicing with me and not YouTube!

If you want to demonstrate something particularly challenging and you decide to do this mid-class, your best option is to ask for help from a student you know and walk them through it. That way, they are supported by supervision, and you can point out the nuances of the practice while they do it, rather than trying to blurt them out while you do it.

Demonstrating is also helpful if someone in your class has hearing loss, deafness, or is practicing yoga in a second language. You may want to encourage them to set up their mat in the middle of the room so they have 360° of visual feedback from other participants. For these students, make a special effort to stand in their line of vision. Reduce other distractions, like loud music, as well.

Also, when I teach chair yoga, I demonstrate the entire class unless I am helping a specific student. There are always exceptional settings and circumstances.

Consider changing the room organization, even if just for an activity.

There is an energetic difference between a mat at the front of the room, the positioning of which says "watch me," compared to a teacher standing as part of a circle with their students while exploring a technique. Standing in a circle conveys the idea, "Let's try it together." When we see each other's faces, when we acknowledge one another's effort and vulnerability, we are co-creating the class as a group.

Journaling Activity

Reach for your journal and reflect on these questions.

When was a time that a teacher demonstrated something and you felt it was really helpful? What were the circumstances? Was it in the flow of practice, or separated out as a "teaching moment"?

What was a time when you felt a teacher's demonstration was distracting to your practice? Did the teacher have other options, or can you think of a reason why they made the choices they did?

Pranayama

WE MAY THINK OF yoga breathing as calming, but to achieve calm, the process may be quite boisterous. *Pranayama* is a practice that can be disruptive. In essence, it disturbs and disrupts our energy, which may have blockages, stagnations, or patterns that are causing suffering or promoting misperception. Yoga practice should shake us up *enough* while simultaneously *providing us with the tools* to cope with what is shaken loose.

The *Hatha Yoga Pradipika* is a medieval era text on yoga practice from which much of Hatha yoga is derived. It says that *pranayama* achieves two aims: it purifies the subtle energy channels called *nadis*, allowing unimpeded *prana* to flow smoothly, making the yogi feel alive and clear. Secondly, *pranayama* draws energy into the central channel of *sushumna,* which effectively dissolves attachments of the ego. In short, it stirs things up internally, but we feel better afterward if we can manage it skillfully—just like a challenging, but beneficial, conversation!

If the practice is *too* provocative, we cannot resolve what comes up in these disruptive practices, and we leave practice disturbed and troubled.

As I remind my students, anything can be provocative. While some *pranayama* practices are specifically meant to be provocative—the *Hatha Yoga Pradipika* outlines one where you stop practice only once you are about to pass out—anything that trains the mind and body can be provocative.

The subtle anatomy perspective on responsible teaching is essential. It is not kind or right to shake people up and plonk them back into their lives, disturbed—there has to be the right practice at the right time, and they need time to wind down. This is part of why we need *Savasana* for integration, but of greater importance: Do not teach overtly provocative practices in group settings. Duration and intensity both play a role in what makes a *pranayama* particularly provocative, so make sure you measure your *pranayama* practices to the appropriate dosage during group classes.

In Patanjali's *Yoga Sutras*, sutra II.52 states that *pranayama* dissolves the "coverings of illumination," which means that it dissolves the ignorance that both overly associates us with the physical realm, and disconnects us from spirit. In many cultures, the breath is linked to life beyond preserving it; it has a more subtle connection to spirit. Consider the French verbs to breathe in and breathe out—*inspirer*, *expirer*—which evolved from the Latin verb for breathing in, *inspirare*, as "in" + *spirare* (spirit). *Spirit moves in, and spirit moves out.*

I have divided the *pranayama* listed here into two sections: Accessible/Calming and Invigorating. This division is perfunctory and debatable, since any practice can be confrontational or provocative, and any yoga practice can be done in a calming or a stimulating manner. Our teaching around *pranayama* should always include a specific disclaimer, "This *pranayama* practice has a calming effect for many people, and you may not find it calming. These are the alternatives...."

If your timing does not often allow alternatives, consider carving out more time for *pranayama*, but always have an alternative for people, such as encouraging them to sit tall and focus on long, slow breathing through the nose (really, the essential practice).

Sitting for Pranayama

Here are a few options for your *pranayama* sit—and they are by no means exhaustive. Since *pranayama* is a practice training us to observe subtleties, we want our sit to be sustainable and not aggravated by insufficient support for your body.

Seated in a Chair (Maitriasana)

Sitting in a chair is an excellent option for both *pranayama* and meditation, particularly if you or your students are unable to get on the ground. Folding chairs are popular for chair yoga because they offer a flat seating surface that easily allows the student to sit upright.

You may want to raise the students' feet up on blocks for more comfort through the hips, stability through the feet and legs, and to promote a sense of grounding.

You may also want to roll a blanket and place it in the small of the back, if the chair has a back.

Seated in a chair is a great place to practice *pranayama* that's more dynamic or detailed because it provides support for the hips and spine. Placing blocks under your feet offers added support for the hips, especially for yogis on the shorter side, whose legs may hang off the chair.

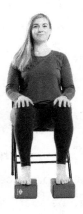

Maitriasana

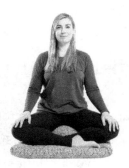

Cross-Legged Sit

Cross-Legged Sit

You can sit raised on a pillow with legs crossed, but resist the urge to tuck your feet into your knees so there are no "kinks in the hose." These practices influence the flow of *prana*, our vital life force, and we want *prana* to flow with ease through its channels, *nadis*, and flow optimally through our circulatory system.

Sitting cross-legged on a meditation cushion, folded blanket, or block provides your hips and spine with needed support. Even if you are a flexible person, demonstrate supported sitting technique when you teach *pranayama*. Otherwise, students may feel they need to mimic you to get the most out of a practice, and they could end up distracted by the effort of holding a seated posture.

Supported Hero (Virasana)

Equally good is sitting on your knees with your hips lifted up on two blocks. There should be lots of support through the pelvis and knees without compression, hence the two blocks stacked up. If you are feeling a moderate stretch through the front of your leg, there is insufficient support.

Stack two blocks with the longest side parallel to the floor (on their widest, shortest setup) on top of each other. You could also place them on a blanket to cushion your knees.

Sit on the blocks so that they land right under your sit bones, with your knees somewhat together and your shins/feet framing the blocks. Sometimes blocks pop out while you're finding a comfortable position—it happens!

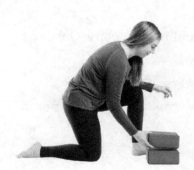 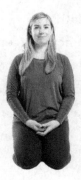

Techniques

Accessible/Calming Pranayama

Dirgha Pranayama (The Long Breath)

The foundational yoga breath is *Dirgha Pranayama*—the long breath. It is commonly called the three-part breath, though I rarely use that term because it promotes a misunderstanding of where we should be focusing our effort in breathing (see the "Breathing" section for more direction).

Dirgha comes from sutra II.52, which states that "pranayama is either outward, or inward, or balanced; it is regulated according to place, time, number; it is protracted and subtle." Since protracted means stretched, this is where we get the "long" breath.

It is the never-ending practice—excellent for beginners and meditation preparation, and should precede all other *pranayama* practice in some amount.

Benefits

- Retrains shallow or anxious breathing patterns by stretching and strengthening the tissues governing breathing
- Promotes a sense of calm and mental clarity by pacifying the nervous system
- Decreases our heart rate and respiratory rate
- Captures our attention and forms the doorway into inner exploration

Cautions and Contraindications

Dirgha Pranayama is usually safe for everyone, but we should use our discretion at all times. If you have a sinus infection or other blockage, this practice may not feel right and it may be best to avoid. If you have experiences of trauma, you never know what can arise in practice. Breath awareness needs to come before pranayama – simply watching breath in a comfortable position is a trauma-sensitive foundation for practice for folks learning to practice pranayama.

Ujjayi Pranayama (Victorious Breath)

Ujjayi (oo-jai-ee) *Pranayama* has been frequently taught during yoga's popularizing era in North America. While popular, few people know the meaning of the word. Most students will think it translates to "oceanic sounding" breath, because that is how it is cued. The word actually translates to "victorious"—victory over death and decay.

I do not often teach *Ujjayi Pranayama* in my classes as part of *asana* practice, because I feel the awareness of how and when to practice fell away as it was habituated in community practice. I have attended and taught classes where *Ujjayi* was "turned on" like a switch was flipped; it seemed to be a sign of "doing the right practice," a sign of attainment.

In my experience, *Ujjayi* forms a "false idol" of *pranayama* practice because of the audible sound that is fairly easy to replicate. Students are able to do it whether or not they have a sound, supple *Dirgha Pranayama* practice.

This is not to blame students for wanting to effectively practice *yoga-asana* and this *pranayama* that often accompanies it. As class lengths have shortened dramatically over the years, many educational elements of class have been cut out. New students sometimes have to rely on observing the behavior of students around them. When the proper application of techniques is not taught, the habit perpetuates.

Teach *Ujjayi!* But teach its proper application with awareness and encourage students to hold every element of practice with reverence.

Benefits

* Audible quality to breath for anchoring practice
* Requires a slowed breathing rate
* Stimulating for the *nadis*, the channels along which *prana* flows
* Warming, very suitable for fall and winter practice

Technique

* *Dirgha pranayama* plus throat restriction – this is a layering technique
* Practice the throat restriction on an exhalation that would fog a mirror
* Then close your lips and replicate it while breathing in and out the nose
* The sound of *Ujjayi* only needs to be audible to the practitioner

Cautions and Contra-indications

Ujjayi Pranayama is safe for most people, but again, it's important that we use our discretion. If you have a sinus infection or other blockage, this may not feel right to you and it may be best not to practice.

Ujjayi should be discouraged for those with chronically high blood pressure, COPD (Chronic Obstructive Pulmonary Disease), or heart disease.

Nadi Shodhana (Channel Purifying Breath)

You likely know *Nadi Shodhana Pranayama* as "alternate nostril breathing." Due to the specificity of the technique and the harmonious pranic flow that it promotes, this *pranayama* is actually "channel purifying breath."

There are a few variations to this one, listed below for you, and they are tremendously beneficial. Swami Kripalu—the Indian sage teacher for whom the yoga center Kripalu was named—was assigned this *pranayama* by his teacher as his only practice for the first year of his yoga journey. It is that potent!

Benefits

* Can be excellent for calming anxiety as it gives the mind an anchor in practice
* Invites an increasingly subtle awareness of our functions, since we may notice disparity from left to right side

- Subtle energy balancing, promotes the harmonious and smooth flow of *prana*

Technique

- There are three parts to this *pranayama*: inhaling through one nostril, retaining (even momentarily), exhaling out the other nostril
- Use right hand to place index and middle finger either to the brow (*Ajna*, third eye *Chakra*) or to palm of hand (*Vishnu mudra*)
  - Switch hands when your hand gets tired, or support your right elbow with your left hand
- Alternatively, use your thumb to block your right nostril, and ring finger and pinkie to block the left nostril, like you were pinching your nose shut one nostril at a time

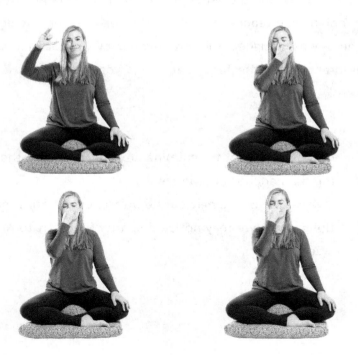

The classic *mudra* for *Nadi Shodhana* is *Vishnu mudra*. Bring your index and middle fingers to the base of the thumb of your right hand and cover your right nostril with your thumb. Alternate covering your nostrils for *Nadi Shodhana*. You can always switch hands and perform *Vishnu mudra* with the other hand!

Variations

- Practice without retention and without the aid of your hand for blocking nostrils (*Anuloma Viloma*)
- Develop even breath (*sama vrtti*) with a breath ration of 4:4:4 to start, and lengthen from there
- Develop uneven breath (*vasama vritti*) with a breath ration of 4:5:6 and lengthen from there

Cautions and Contraindications

For yogis with circulatory or heart disease, pregnant women, or those with high anxiety, we do not recommend breath retention.

When teaching any *pranayama*, remind yogis that even practices that can be calming for *many* people can be anxiety-inducing for *some* people. Especially with breath rationing or retention, this is particularly contra-indicated for trauma-sensitive classes.

Brahmari (Bee/Buzzing Breath)

In Hindu mythology, there was a terrible demon named Arunasura, who was impervious to being killed, because he had managed to get a boon (favor) from Brahma by standing on one leg and chanting sacred verses for a few thousand years.

The boon he asked for prevented him from being killed by a two- or four-legged creature, any man or woman, and in any manner of war. With his power, he ran amok, challenging the gods (*devas*) and wreaking havoc.

The goddess Shakti was embodied in physical form (*rupa*) as Brahmari, who was able to command insects, from spiders to bees. With this ability, she called a great swarm of bees to her aid, and Arunasura was defeated. Brahmari is remembered as the goddess of the bees, and this *pranayama* is named for her because of the buzzing sound it produces. May our practice of *brahmari* help us be as creative as she!

Because of the gentle warming and introversion of this *pranayama*, it is an excellent *pranayama* for fall and wintertime.

Benefits

- Calms and quiets the mind; can be quite soothing
- Promotes release of mental tension
- Is said to support the pituitary gland functioning, which is the "master gland" that dictates many physiological functions
- Cultivates a sense of introversion and inner awareness

Technique

- Breathe in and out through the nose
- Full inhalation through the nose like *Dirgha Pranayama*, exhalation through the nose, making a buzzing noise
- Think of humming the letter "M"

* *Khechari mudra*: flip the tip of the tongue to the soft palette of the mouth *only* on exhalation to channel the energy upward—"shaking the cobwebs" loose

Variations

* *Pratyahara*: cover the ears with thumbs and lay the index and middle finger lightly over the eyes
* *Shanmukhi mudra*: one thumb on each tragus (triangular ear covering), index fingers lightly covering eyelids near the inside corners, the middle fingers on the sides of the nose, ring fingers and pinkies framing the lips above and below
* Experiment with pitch and notice the qualities (*gunas)* it cultivates
* *Brahmari* can be a lovely addition to the closing of a class or in more introverted postures, like forward folds toward the end of class—try incorporating three rounds of this *pranayama*. It helps transition the class from sound to quiet.

Cautions and Contraindications

While *Brahmari* is a widely accessible *pranayama*, always use your discretion. It is not appropriate if you have a sinus infection or nasal passage obstruction.

Invigorating Pranayama

Kapalabhati Pranayama (Shining Skull Breath)

Some people know this pranayama as "breath of fire," but in the Hatha yoga tradition, it is Shining Skull Breath. This particular *pranayama* and the one below, *Bhastrika*, are both excellent *pranayama* for springtime because of the influence of earth and water elements. During springtime, we are more likely to be depressed and lethargic because of the heaviness of the season. Sharp, strong, hot practices like these two *pranayama* can be motivating and invigorating for such a time.

Benefits

- Warming and invigorating
- Gives one a "steadiness at center" before moving into other practice or continuing your day
- Breaks up feelings of sluggishness and heaviness, promoting flow of *prana*
- Improves digestive fire (*agni*)

Technique

- Vigorous exhalations followed by passive inhalations— imagine a cough action, or blowing out a candle with your nose
- Primary movement from the belly, like you were trying to "snap" the belly button back toward the spine
- Hands rest on your thighs or knees and stay relaxed
- Relax the shoulders

- Try 20–30 exhalations and see how you feel, allow it to integrate before moving on
- Then try an additional 30–40 exhalations if 30 felt achievable
- In a typical class, the average person will not feel they need to exceed 40
- Offer this practice in one or two rounds and give one minute for integration

Cautions and Contraindications

These cautions are the same for *Kapalabhati* as they are for *Bhastrika*.

These exciting *pranayama* are not appropriate for anyone with heart disease, COPD, chronic high blood pressure, hernias, ulcers, spinal injuries, or those who are pregnant, who have recently had surgery, or who suffer from mental/emotional instability. The earlier notes on sinus infection apply too.

Students who are menstruating may not want to practice *Kapalabhati*, as it stimulates the downward flow of energy *(apana vayu)*.

Please take special note of and remember to teach the contraindication of mental/emotional instability, as these are powerful practices that require a bodymind stable enough to practice them. We do not want to further destabilize containers.

You also need to set the pace for *Kapalabhati*, as students who are familiar with the technique, but confuse rapidity for achievement, will excite the room.

Bhastrika (Bellows Breath)

If *Kapalabhati* is vigorous in one direction, *Bhastrika* is vigorous in both. I rarely teach this *pranayama* in drop-in classes, but I have worked it into classes when I know everyone in the room and have a familiarity with their practice. I use it in my own practice when I want a dramatic experience of moving *prana*. Remember though, we want *prana* to flow smoothly, not erratically. If you are feeling erratic or overly exerted, it is not the right time for *Bhastrika*.

Both *Kapalabhati* and *Bhastrika* require warmup with a few minutes of *Dirgha Pranayama* and/or warming *asana*.

Benefits

- ◆ Energizing and clarifying breath
- ◆ Also excellent for springtime
- ◆ Very stimulating (not recommended before bedtime)

Technique

- ◆ Strong inhalation and exhalation of equal length
- ◆ Exaggerating thoracic movement with short, sharp breaths
- ◆ Allow your body to go with the movement, some rocking around your seat is normal
- ◆ Try 20–30 exhalations and see how you feel, allow it to integrate while you quietly observe
- ◆ Then try an additional 30–40 exhalations if 30 felt achievable
- ◆ In a typical class, the average person will not feel they need to exceed 40

* Offer it in one or two rounds and give at least one minute for integration

Variation

* Arm movements: reaching up with fingers extended as you inhale, closing fists and bringing hands down to shoulders on exhalation, kind of like a "fist pump"
* Arm movement variation: reaching forward with wide fingers, closing fists and bringing hands down to tuck to sides with exhalations
* Hands to belly
* One hand to belly, one hand to lower back

Teaching Pranayama

Pranayama is an incredible practice that hones the mind-body connection, strengthens complex musculature through the torso, cultivates specific energetic outcomes, and is an excellent preparation for meditation.

Yet, many yogis do not have a consistent *pranayama* practice, and there is a tendency in modern yoga culture to only layer it on top of the *asana* practice, not breaking it out as its own activity.

A regular *pranayama* practice is a gift, and requires less space and set up than *asana*. Just like *asana*, however, the practice should be attuned to the practitioner's skillfulness and the seasons. *How* we do something is as important as *what* we do.

Below are specific guidelines to teaching *pranayama* when students have little to no familiarity with the practice. I do not always follow every step outlined below when teaching *pranayama*, but I do ask my trainees to go through each step specifically. Learning how to teach a specific sequence of instructions will make it easier to teach fluidly in the future as you turn the sequence into a habit.

Steps to Teaching Pranayama

1. Describe and demonstrate how to sit for *pranayama* practice and allow time for adjustments
2. Introduce the *pranayama* with its Sanskrit name, common name, and translation
3. Share one or two of the benefits of the *pranayama*
4. Provide "yellow light" cautions—undesirable effects that could happen
5. Provide "red light" contraindications—who should not be practicing and what their alternative options could be
6. Describe the process
7. Demonstrate the *pranayama*
8. Invite students to practice one round
9. Clarify and answer questions
10. Lead a longer, more experiential round and offer any additional technique details toward the beginning
11. Allow for absorption and reflection

Example:

1 + 2. *Establish your seat for our* Nadi Shodhana, *or Alternate Nostril Breath,* pranayama *practice. You can sit raised on a pillow with legs crossed, but resist the urge to tuck your feet into your knees so there are no "kinks in the hose." We want* prana *to flow with ease through its channels. Equally good is sitting on your knees with your hips lifted up on two blocks. There should be lots of support through the pelvis and knees, without feeling any compression.*

3. *This is my favorite practice in preparation for meditation, and it is pacifying to the mind and nervous system.*

4. *If you have sinus congestion, you may be uncomfortable in this particular* pranayama, *but you're welcome to try and see how it goes.*

5. *This* pranayama *is safe for most of us, but should not be practiced by anyone with a deviated septum. Many people find this* pranayama *focusing and calming, but occasionally folks find it aggravating. You are welcome to try it and then return to the beneficial four square breathing we typically do.*

6. *To focus the mind on the breath practice, we use our hand to block one nostril while we breathe through the other, so air can flow evenly and rhythmically through one nostril at a time. You can go to two-thirds or full breath capacity. You can also support the elbow of your* mudra *arm with your other hand if it gets tired.*

7. *This is what it looks like.* (Demonstrate *mudra*, support, and *pranayama* for two rounds.)

8. *Tuck your fingers into* Vishnu mudra *by placing your index and middle fingers to the base of your thumb. Cover your right nostril with your thumb and exhale all air out through the left, then slowly breathe in through your left nostril. Cover your left nostril and exhale out your right, then slowly inhale through your right, cover, and exhale out the left. Continue for two minutes.*

9. *Exhale out your left nostril and then breathe evenly through both. Notice what you feel—there's no right or wrong answer. Flutter open your eyes. Are there any questions?*

10. *Get comfortable, tuck your fingers back into* Vishnu mudra, *and this time we'll practice quietly for a few minutes...relax your eyes... remember that this grows easier with experience, and it's already beneficial...soften your belly and continue.*

11. *Relax both hands onto your knees. Breathe evenly through both nostrils. Notice the qualities of your mind. Now mindfully come down onto your back...*

Planning Classes

THE ELEMENTS OF YOUR class that you choose to plan will depend on where you are teaching, if you have the same or varying studentship (drop-in or pre-registered), and how your class is described and advertised to students.

You can plan a loose class structure around a theme. With teaching experience you grow an understanding of how to choreograph short sequences that work for your desired outcome, be it atmosphere, attentiveness, preparation for a progressive postures, etc. You will develop an understanding of sequencing a class as a whole to suit your students' needs as you learn about the people you are teaching with repeat attendance. Planning can be a critical element of teaching well, since you can offer more philosophy, *pranayama*, and meditation or guided relaxation. Many teachers find class themes a suitably cohesive anchor—like an essay's thesis, all components are working toward its realization.

Sometimes, when I was feeling keen to teach a long and thorough sequence, my plans felt dashed. I may know a class quite well, but a student may have an injury to accommodate, or someone is attending their first class ever. I remember planning an arm balance sequence, only to have a student show up to say, "I sprained my wrist and I knew you could still teach without much wrist stuff." Of course I was going to honor their time and trust required to show up that evening.

Many wise teachers have said it: *teach to who shows up.* Learning how to teach without a plan takes a lot of planning and practice, but it is within your reach. On the occasions when you know your group and they show up ready to go, enjoy the rarity of it all going according to plan. This is the essence of our practice and our teaching: prepare, *and* prepare to let go.

Feeling More Confident

If you decide to teach yoga, you will find that teaching is far less intimidating out in the world than in your yoga teacher training. There will be no experienced mentor sitting at the back of the room, comparing your class against a rubric! Still, whether you are new to teaching or find yourself teaching in a higher-stakes environment—like a new studio, or a corporate lunch gig—rely on these tips to improve your confidence.

Develop an accessible, well-rounded sequence that is your "go to." There is nothing wrong with repeating the same sequence in different classes! Also, if people are only practicing once a week, then doing the same sequence weekly with minor variations is still very good for their bodies. A calm, clear, plain yoga class is a superior experience to a confusing, but novel, one.

Know your mini-sequences. These are useful to memorize so that you can create sequences easily by essentially grouping many mini-sequences together. One of my assistants referred to it as "chunking" your sequences—the overall class comes together by linking different chunks.

Develop a theme. A theme can anchor your talks, your readings, and your postures in your classes.

Develop a class series. Depending on your teaching setting, you may be able to develop a six-class series that is pre-planned. You could do different themes each week, and those could be postural, or more thematic. This allows you to pre-plan without feeling repetitive, plus you get to know your students. These series can be rewarding for teachers and students, including being more financially sustainable for yoga teachers.

Make sure you practice. The best way to know what to teach is to experiment on your own yoga mat. Stay inspired by taking led classes from teachers you enjoy, and try new teachers in the spirit of diversity and discovery.

Sample Class Themes

<u>*Autumn Equinox*</u>

Opening Talk

- Whether you are sad to see summer wane or excited for the coming holidays, autumn is a season of transition that wakes us up to the passage of time.
- A season of change—a sense of movement and turning over—invites nostalgia and reflection.
- The reflectiveness of the season and the bounty of the harvest is ripe for gratitude practice.
- Ayurveda tells us that the qualities of the coming season begin to accumulate in the season before, so if we do not prepare for winter, we're already behind the curve when it arrives.
- In the spirit of preparation, we're going to do a steady, rhythmic class that moderately harnesses the vitality of summer, with a long class wind-down that feels like a cozy entry to hibernation.

Asana **sequence**: Begin slowly, responding to felt sensations and initiating movement from breath, alternate between steady core work and rooted standing postures like Warrior I and II, moving toward an introverted cooldown with two well-propped forward folds.

Pranayama: *Anuloma Viloma* to cultivate a gentle focus.

Closing reading: Mary Oliver's poem *Wild Geese*.

<u>Building Confidence</u>

Opening Talk

- The Buddhist teacher Jack Kornfield tells a story about how, at a summit of Buddhists, the Eastern Buddhist teachers, including the Dalai Lama, couldn't understand the Western teachers saying that "self-loathing" was a problem for Western students. It took 10 minutes for his translator to convey the concept, to which the Dalai Lama said, "But don't they know they're precious?!"
- Many of us struggle with a lack of confidence, and to-day's practice is intended to cultivate self-compassion as well as steadiness, in our wisdom and ourselves.
- Offer an intention/affirmation and have them repeat it to themselves silently, such as:
  - My heart is wise
  - I have a voice worth hearing
  - I stand firmly in my strength
  - I am precious

Asana **sequence**: A practice that moves between cultivating intuitive movement (i.e., not "rules-y" alignment postures) and poses with expressive arms—"power poses." Releasing tension through the ribcage through standing backbends, seated side bends, etc. Slow wind down with feel-good postures and lots of prop support.

Pranayama: *Dirgha Pranayama* to warm up breathing, 2 x 20 steady, warming rounds of *Kapalabhati*, end with two minutes of reflective *Dirgha Pranayama* to integrate.

Closing reading: A passage from Tara Brach's *Radical Acceptance.*

Scope of Practice for a Yoga Teacher

A "scope of practice" refers to the activities that particular certifications, educations, or professions permit you to do. The term "yoga teacher" includes a lot of people with varying skillfulness and experience, so I felt it might be helpful to guide us toward right action by considering the scope of practice of a yoga teacher.

Considering how to live our yoga includes using the ethical guidelines of yoga to guide our behavior. What constitutes ethical conduct is not easy or obvious to determine, which is why every generation produces its own moral philosophers.

When you first read about the concept of *satya*, or truthfulness, you may think it is easy—simply do not lie. However, exaggeration is a form of non-truthfulness. When we exaggerate, our speech is not even (*sama)*, but imbalanced.

Studies show varying quantities of lies in our daily interactions. Why do we lie, especially when in neutral situations? It is an attempt to amplify how we are received—through exaggeration and falsehoods, we hope to shape how others see us.

Dr. David Livingstone-Smith, a professor at the Institute for Cognitive Psychology at the University of New England, studies why people lie to each other and themselves (self-deception). He outlines how deception is an adaptive trait to influence

TEACH KIND, CLEAR YOGA

how we see ourselves and how others see us; we mostly deceive casually.

Livingstone-Smith says that some self-deception is necessary for survival, but that we can get rid of "excess" deceit by cultivating self-awareness. A critical component of this is learning to be comfortable with identifying our desires and motivations, and being kind to ourselves in interactions.

Depending on your experience in other fields and your natural talents, students do not always appreciate the scope of practice for a teacher. I recall a time in my first year of teaching when a young woman had a back injury that made *Savasana* uncomfortable. I offered her some options for making her *Savasana* more comfortable, and encouraged her to experiment with them—this was within my scope of practice.

After class, we started chatting about the back injury and I casually started suggesting other exercises for alleviating pain—outside my scope of practice. It turned out that I knew this person through another friend, and her back injury was in fact far more severe than she had let on. While she ultimately overcame the injury, it was through a combination of yoga practice and physical therapy, tailored to specifically address her needs.

Similarly, I have yoga teacher training graduates admit to me that students ask them questions about troublesome or advanced yoga postures, and they "come up with something" in the moment.

The urge to help people asking us for help is strong. We may say to ourselves that we are trying to be of service; however, I think we need to acknowledge the strong pull toward satisfying our ego by providing an answer.

When you graduate yoga teacher training, you can lead a yoga class! That is a great and sufficient offering, and we can let group yoga classes stand in their strength as an excellent practice for most people and an excellent adjunct practice for people pursuing therapy for a specific need.

Within the scope of your practice, one of the best courses of action is learning to adapt and change yoga postures. This begins with the question: "What happens when you...?" You and your student will collaboratively identify a pain-free space to be in, and you can also help them identify the differences in movements that cause pain so that when they see their manual therapist, they have more information to share.

Remember to Refer Out

Reading and taking continuing education courses are helpful resources, but understanding moving bodies takes time and observation. I feel that graduates of my teacher training program are well-equipped to facilitate a yoga class. Still, I encourage them to "refer out" for specific questions, even to other yoga teachers.

More experienced yoga teachers are great resources for specific needs. I am always sharing these "resources" with my students: *Oh, Mike is great if you want to learn a handstand! Yes, my friend Erin specializes in yoga for chronic pain—get your phone and I will give you her website.*

I always carry cards for psychotherapists and physical therapists, and happily pass on all sorts of recommendations to other teachers. It is right to be honest about your scope of knowledge; it is another practice of seeing ourselves as students first. The culture of referral is a good one to support.

Sure, you may position yourself as a newer teacher, but you will also position yourself as someone who is honest, genuinely concerned about that person's wellness and safety, a student of yoga yourself, and someone with a trustworthy network.

To build faith with yourself (your most important relationship!) others, and your students, you have to begin with truth-telling in your speech.

Journaling Activity

For one day, carry a journal and a pen with you throughout your normal day. Observe yourself in conversations and reflect afterward with these questions.

Did the situation make you anxious, and you withheld or changed the truth to alleviate that anxiety? What didn't feel safe or calm about the exchange?

Did your conversant have something valuable (status, influence), pushing you to engage in self-deception or deception to influence how they saw you?

Do some relationships feel like they rely on superficial depth or omission to maintain harmony?

Building Each Other Up

As so many of us strive to carve a path in the yogic realm that is intellectually, spiritually, and financially sustainable, it can feel challenging to be generous-of-spirit with other yogis. We see that someone else seems successful, and feel that their success is bad for our business.

In the early portion of the book on the *Yoga Sutras*, I mentioned that there were probably "Patanjalis"; that he is more of a mythical figure, and multiple yogis attributed their work to this sage. What a contrast to the modern era, where everyone is developing a method or trademark!

When we are doing our *dharma* talks, posting to social media, etc., it is a beautiful practice to build each other up and form a network, rather than remain an island. Sharing yogis, thinkers, activists, and teachers who inspire us, or where we heard ideas, is less about acknowledging trademarks, and more about recognizing the diversity of wise voices out there.

Learning from Other Classes and Teachers

Once you begin yoga teacher training, class experiences change for you. You now assess the class structure, listen to cues differently, and are aware of the sequencing—you may even be internally distracted by questions and analyses during class.

In my yoga teacher trainings, the homework assignments include attending a diversity of classes. It is so refreshing to see how differently people interpret yoga—especially when you seek out classes with different emphases and intended audiences.

The exercise is not to judge the merits of other teachers, but to learn about class structure, yoga space culture, how teachers share their knowledge, etc. I encourage trainees to journal and analyze with the same compassion you would like future teachers in training to bring to your classes!

Above all, consider why someone may be doing something the way they are—there are many reasons people make their offerings, and some are not observable as a participant.

Sometimes the yoga space has regulations they have to follow, sometimes the season of their own life seeps into their teaching, or they are merely addressing the needs and wants of the people who consistently show up. Think about that when you practice: What is it that appeals to people here? Most successful studios and classes strike a balance between offerings that are popular and "keep the lights on," and practices that perhaps cultivate a richer experience of yoga.

First of all, when you attend classes, do a self-check to see if you need time away from teaching method analysis. It could just be another internal distraction that you need to set aside. If you are feeling sufficiently balanced and supported in your practice though, consider the following questions.

- How was the class structured—in time, physical space, setup, etc.?
- Did the teacher begin class with a talk?
- Were you acknowledged by the teacher?

- Were there props used—encouraged, or simply available for use? How did the teacher describe prop use?
- How did the teacher approach their teaching—off the mat, hands-on, demonstrative?
- What elements did the teacher employ for atmosphere in the class—music, lights, scents, etc.?
- What cues did the teacher use that resonated with you?
- What do you know of this style's lineage ahead of the class, and how did the class line up with or diverge from this knowledge?
- What postures were new/surprising for you?
- What sequencing felt good in your bodymind, and why do you think it worked for you (familiarity, novelty, alignment of your needs today, etc.)?
- What sequencing didn't make sense for your bodymind and why?

Beginner Courses

Occasionally, I still attend Beginner Meditation or Yoga 101 workshops from time to time to see how other teachers facilitate for every level of experience. When I attend a training session, I still pay attention, even when I think, *I know this stuff already.* There is always something to be learned from how facilitators manage their training, and there is a lot of information in the structure. If you move into the realm of facilitating special classes and workshops, consider these questions in assessing other teachers' work.

- How did the teacher handle questions? Were they saved for the end of class, or responded to throughout?
- How much of the program was lecture, and how much was experiential?
- Were the handouts thorough or vague, and did that support or hinder the experiential components of the program?
- How did the teacher manage group work? Partner work?
- How do you think the number of people in the room influenced their programming choices?
- What was it about the facilitator that you found effective? Did they honor the timing and schedule of the program?

Conclusion

WHEN MY SON WAS born, I developed a terrible anxiety any time he was near knives. He was still a babe-in-arms, but his vulnerability, coupled with the pressure of new parenthood, resulted in this irrational fear. At the same time, I recognized that birth is an incredible feat of physical endurance for mom and baby.

In learning to cope with this fear, I developed an affirmation: *Human life is both fragile and resilient.* It reminded me that some fear was helpful motivation to create a safe home and parent mindfully, but it also reminded me that humans are resilient beings. Life is both precious and enduring.

Becoming a parent underscored what I already knew as a yoga teacher. If you teach yoga and learn about how people move, contemplate, rest, and assimilate the teachings of yoga into their lives, you will also be struck by how fragile *and* resilient bodyminds can be.

The fragility of the bodymind will inspire you to be thoughtful and humble in your offerings; to continuously refine your methods and take into account new information and other interpretations or perspectives.

The resilience of the bodymind will remind you that yoga has something to offer anyone interested in trying it, and as long as the effort is scaled to their needs, they will appreciate the transformative powers of yoga as you do.

While I described yoga as a science at the beginning of the book, we explored many aspects of practice and teaching that center on the artistry inherent in yoga. Both scientists and artists refine their methods over time, as I hope you will, too. I hope you have discovered some tools of artistry and science in this book for improving the accessibility of your classes, and for teaching with greater clarity. Widening the circle of yoga and teaching with a compassionate lens *is* available to you.

I wish you all the best on this path of refinement, this yoga.

Gratitude

WHENEVER IT COMES TIME to express gratitude for a community gathering, it's an opportunity to acknowledge our interconnectedness - to recognize the many people who contributed to making it possible. When one begins to ask – who has helped me arrive here? – the practice goes deep and wide.

Thank you to Alex, my root system and my love. And to Harvey, who is helping me hone my yoga all the time.

Thank you to my parents; you are my first and forever teachers.

To Mona. Thank you for multiple rounds of feedback and encouragement and for an almost equal ratio of smiley faces to question marks in your markups. You and your teaching are blessings to many.

Thank you to Melissa McLean, Dr. Geoff Outerbridge, Janine Clarke, and Dr. Jennifer Musial for your wisdom, clarifications, and feedback.

Thank you to Ro Nwosu and Carly Stong, my *asana* models.

Thank you to my editor, Lesley-Anne Longo, for wielding your editorial "sword of compassion" with precision.

Thank you to Amanda, my helper friend, for your discernment and diligence.

Thank you to Nicole for your artistry and your grace-under-email.

Thank you to Sophie for your proofreading and gentle nudges toward clarity.

Thank you to Elena for encouraging me to do this in the first place.

Thank you to Michael, who is so missed and whose teachings infuse my daily practice with direction.

To my students, thank you for being my source and my outlet. I think of you more than you may realize; you occupy such real estate in my heart and head.

References

1   Tapper, J. (2013, March 19). Yoga's evolution: From basement studios to big business. The Toronto Star. https://www.thestar.com/life/health_wellness/fitness/2013/03/19/yogas_evolution_from_basement_studios_to_big_business.html

2   Statistics Canada. (n.d.). High blood pressure by age group. https://www150.statcan.gc.ca/t1/tbl1/en/tv.action?pid=1310009609

3   Statistics Canada. (2019, June 25). Overweight and obese adults by age group. https://www150.statcan.gc.ca/n1/pub/82-625-x/2019001/article/00005-eng.htm

4   Barden, M., & Morgon, A. (2015). A beautiful constraint: How to transform your limitations into advantages, and why it's everyone's business. Wiley.

5   White, D. G. (2019). The yoga sutra of Patanjali: A biography. Princeton University Press.

6   Feuerstein, G. (2003). What you may not realize about yoga. Yoga International. https://yogainternational.com/article/view/what-you-may-not-realize-about-yoga/

7   Duhigg, C. (2014). The power of habit: Why we do what we do in life and business. Random House.

8   Raveh, D. (2016). Sūtras, stories and yoga philosophy: Narrative and transfiguration. Routledge.

9   Phillip, M. (2019, March 5). Even with a Harvard pedigree, caste follows like a shadow. PRI. https://www.pri.org/stories/2019-03-05/even-harvard-pedigree-caste-follows-shadow

10   Wildcroft, T. (2020, January 28). Separate the teachings from the teacher. Wild Yoga. https://www.wildyoga.co.uk/2020/01/separate-the-teacher-from-the-teachings/

11   Sparrowe, L. (2014). Transcending trauma: How yoga heals. Yoga International. https://yogainternational.com/article/view/transcending-trauma-how-yoga-heals

12   Easwaran, E., & Nagler, M.N. (1987). The Upanishads. Petaluma, CA: Nilgiri Press.

13   Carnegie Mellon University. (n.d.) Benefits of self-affirmation. https://www.cmu.edu/homepage/health/2013/summer/benefits-of-self-affirmations.html

14   Ariely, D. (2009). Our buggy moral code [Video]. TED. https://www.ted.com/talks/dan_ariely_our_buggy_moral_code/transcript?language=en

15   Cloer, D. (2004). The synaptic connection. Vision. http://www.vision.org/visionmedia/article.aspx%3Fid%3D321

16   Patañjali, & Hartranft, C. (2003). The Yoga-Sūtra of Patañjali: A new translation with commentary. Shambhala Publications.

17   Doidge, N. (2007). The brain that changes itself: Stories of personal triumph from the frontiers of brain science. Penguin Books.

18   Pascual-Leone, A., Amedi, A., Fregni, F., & Merabet, L. B. (2005). The plastic human brain cortex. Annual Review of Neuroscience, 28, 377–401. https://doi: 10.1146/ annurev.neuro.27.070203.144216

19   Pascual-Leone, A. (2016, May 16). How to keep your brain healthy with exercise. [Video]. Harvard Health Publishing. https://www.youtube.com/watch?v=VUSIVuXiWUo

20   Hargrove, T. (2008, September 12). How to improve proprioception. Better Movement. https://www.bettermovement.org/blog/2008/proprioception-the-3-d-map-of-the-body

21   Ager, A., Borms, D., Deschepper, L., Dhooghe, R., Dijkhuis, J.,Roy, J.S., & Cools, A. (2019). Proprioception: How is it affected by shoulder pain? A systematic review. Journal of Hand Therapy. https://10.1016/j.jht.2019.06.002.

22   Hargrove, T. (2008, September 12). How to improve proprioception. Better Movement. https://www.bettermovement.org/blog/2008/proprioception-the-3-d-map-of-the-body

23   Baliki, M. N., & Apkarian, A. V. (2015). Nociception, pain, negative moods, and behavior selection. Neuron, 87(3), 474–491. https://doi.org/10.1016/j.neuron.2015.06.005

24   Krans, J. L. (2010). The sliding filament theory of muscle contraction. Nature Education, 3(9), 66.

25   Connor, P. M., Banks, D. M., Tyson, A. B., Coumas, J. S., & D'Alessandro, D. F. (2003). Magnetic resonance imaging of the asymptomatic shoulder of overhead athletes: A 5-year follow-up study. The American Journal of Sports Medicine, 31(5), 724–727. https://doi.org/10.1177/03635465030310051501

26   Harvard Health Letter. (2010). You've torn your ACL. now what? Harvard Medical School. https://www.health.harvard.edu/newsletter_article/youve-torn-your-acl-now-what

27   Lee, D. (2016, September 15). Clinical specialist Diane Lee on why women's health is more than the pelvic floor. Canadian Physiotherapy Association. https://physiotherapy.ca/blog/clinical-specialist-diane-lee-why-womens-health-more-pelvic-floor

28   Gatchel, R. J., & Krista, J. H. (2018). The biopsychosocial approach. Practical Pain Management Journal, 8(4). https://www.practicalpainmanagement.com/treatments/psychological/biopsychosocial-approach

29   Kaminoff, L., & Matthews, A. (2011).Yoga anatomy (2nd ed.). Human Kinetics.

30   Thomas, B. (2015, February 2). Dr. Stephen Levin: Biotensegrity. [Audio podcast episode]. In Liberated Body podcast. Liberated Body. https://www.liberatedbody.com/podcast/stephen-levin-lbp-035

31   Flynn, K. (2018, March 18). Fascia, anatomy and movement with Joanne Sarah Avison. [Audio podcast episode]. In intelligent edge yoga podcast. Intelligent edge yoga. http://intelligentedge.yoga/journal/2018/3/18/podcast-ep-13-fascia-anatomy-and-movement-with-joanne-sarah-avison

32   Rawlings, J. (2017). Fascia myths and fascia facts. Yoga International. https://yogainternational.com/article/view/fascia-myths-and-fascia-facts

33   Schoenfeld, B. J. (2010). The mechanisms of muscle hypertrophy and their application to resistance training. Journal of Strength and Conditioning Research, 24(10), 2857–2872. https://doi.org/10.1519/jsc.0b013e3181e840f3

34   van der Waal, J. (2013). Proprioception. In R. Schleip, T. W. Findley, L. Chaitow, & P. A. Huijing (Eds.), Fascia: The tensional network of the human body (pp. 81–88). Elsevier.

35   Schleip, R. & Jager, H. (2013). Interoception: A new correlate for intricate connections between fascial receptors, emotion, and self recognition. In R. Schleip, T. W. Findley, L. Chaitow, & P. A. Huijing (Eds.), Fascia: The tensional network of the human body (pp. 89–94). Elsevier.

36   Blakeslee, S., & Blakeslee, M. (2008). The body has a mind of its own: How body maps in your brain help you do (almost) everything better. Random House.

37   Blakeslee, S., & Blakeslee, M. (2008). The body has a mind of its own: How body maps in your brain help you do (almost) everything better. Random House.

38   Pascual-Leone A., & Torres, F. (1993). Plasticity of the sensorimotor cortex representation of the reading finger in Braille readers. Brain, 116(1), 39–52.

39   Singleton, M. (2010).Yoga body: The origins of modern posture practice. Oxford University Press.

40   Johansson, T., & Andreasson, J. (2016). The gym and the beach: Globalization, situated bodies, and Australian fitness. Journal of Contemporary Ethnography, 45(2), 143–167. https://doi.org/10.1177/0891241614554086

41   Singleton, M. (2010).Yoga body: The origins of modern posture practice. Oxford University Press.

42   Remski, M. (2018, April 25). Yoga's culture of sexual abuse. The Walrus. https://thewalrus.ca/yogas-culture-of-sexual-abuse-nine-women-tell-their-stories/

About the Author

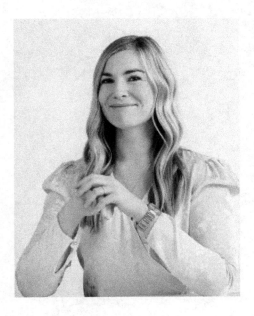

KATHRYN ANNE FLYNN IS a teacher and student of yoga, meditation, and Ayurveda in Ottawa, Canada, where she is completing her Masters in Clinical Psychotherapy. Recognized for her articulate and thoughtful voice, Kathryn is known for weaving together her fields of study and practice tools to meet life with a compassionate presence. Students of many generations call her their teacher, drawn to her inclusivity and authenticity.

You can listen to her podcast, practice with her online, and find out about upcoming training, workshops, and retreats at www.kathrynanneflynn.com.

CPSIA information can be obtained
at www.ICGtesting.com
Printed in the USA
LVHW081523120621
690063LV00003B/303